PUBLIC HEALTH IN THE 21ST CENTURY

Additional books in this series can be found on Nova's website under the Series tab.

Additional E-books in this series can be found on Nova's website under the E-books tab.

PUBLIC HEALTH IN THE 21ST CENTURY

HERNIAS

TYPES, SYMPTOMS AND TREATMENT

JAMES H. WAGNER
EDITOR

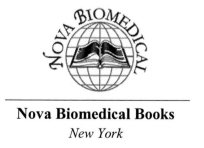

Nova Biomedical Books
New York

Copyright © 2011 by Nova Science Publishers, Inc.

All rights reserved. No part of this book may be reproduced, stored in a retrieval system or transmitted in any form or by any means: electronic, electrostatic, magnetic, tape, mechanical photocopying, recording or otherwise without the written permission of the Publisher.

For permission to use material from this book please contact us:
Telephone 631-231-7269; Fax 631-231-8175
Web Site: http://www.novapublishers.com

NOTICE TO THE READER

The Publisher has taken reasonable care in the preparation of this book, but makes no expressed or implied warranty of any kind and assumes no responsibility for any errors or omissions. No liability is assumed for incidental or consequential damages in connection with or arising out of information contained in this book. The Publisher shall not be liable for any special, consequential, or exemplary damages resulting, in whole or in part, from the readers' use of, or reliance upon, this material. Any parts of this book based on government reports are so indicated and copyright is claimed for those parts to the extent applicable to compilations of such works.

Independent verification should be sought for any data, advice or recommendations contained in this book. In addition, no responsibility is assumed by the publisher for any injury and/or damage to persons or property arising from any methods, products, instructions, ideas or otherwise contained in this publication.

This publication is designed to provide accurate and authoritative information with regard to the subject matter covered herein. It is sold with the clear understanding that the Publisher is not engaged in rendering legal or any other professional services. If legal or any other expert assistance is required, the services of a competent person should be sought. FROM A DECLARATION OF PARTICIPANTS JOINTLY ADOPTED BY A COMMITTEE OF THE AMERICAN BAR ASSOCIATION AND A COMMITTEE OF PUBLISHERS.

Additional color graphics may be available in the e-book version of this book.

Library of Congress Cataloging-in-Publication Data
Hernias : types, symptoms, and treatment / editor, James H. Wagner.
   p. ; cm.
   Includes bibliographical references and index.
   ISBN 978-1-61324-125-7 (hardcover : alk. paper) 1. Hernia--Surgery. I. Wagner, James H. (James Herbert), 1964-
   [DNLM: 1. Hernia--surgery. 2. Hernia--diagnosis. WI 950]
   RD621.H49 2011
   617.5'59059--dc22
                                                                                                    2011007922

Published by Nova Science Publishers, Inc. ✦ New York

Contents

Preface vii

Chapter 1 Minimally Invasive Repair of Inguinal
Hernias in Children 1
Hiotshi Ikeda

Chapter 2 Surgical Approach to Parastomal Hernias 31
*V.B. Tsirline, I. Belyansky, D.A. Klima, K.L. Harold
and B.T. Heniford*

Chapter 3 Hernias: Types, Symptoms and Treatment 57
Ho-Hsing Lin and Chi-Wen Juan

Chapter 4 Impact of Prophylactic Fundoplication on Survival
without Growth Disorder in Left Congenital
Diaphragmatic Hernias Requiring a Patch Repair 81
*Anne Dariel, Jean-Christophe Roze,
Hugues Piloquet, G. Podevin
and the French CDH Study Group*

Chapter 5 Hiatal Hernias: Classification,
Pathophysiology and Treatment 99
*Lourdes Robles, Christopher S. Davis and
P. Marco Fisichella*

Chapter 6	The Applicability, Alternation and Future Research in Laparoscopic Surgery for Pediatric Inguinal Hernias *Yu-Tang Chang*	111
Chapter 7	Incidence and Risk Factors for an Incisional Hernia after Severe Secondary Peritonitis *Pascal Jeanmonod, Sven Richter, Jochen Schuld, Christoph Justinger, Otto Kollmar, Martin K. Schilling and Mohammed R. Moussavian*	125
Chapter 8	Surgical Approach to Umbilical Hernias: Then and Now *Igor Belyansky, Victor B. Tsirline, David A. Klima, Ronald F. Sing and B. Todd Heniford*	139
Chapter 9	Eventration Disease of the Abdominal Wall *Andrew A. Gassman, Anupama Mehta, Casey Thomas and P. Marco Fisichella*	161
Chapter 10	Spigelian Hernias *David A. Klima, Igor Belyansky, Victor B. Tsirline and B. Todd Heniford*	191
Index		207

Preface

A hernia is the protrusion of an organ or the fascia of an organ through the wall of the cavity that normally contains it. A hiatal hernia occurs when the stomach protrudes into the mediastinum through the esophageal opening in the diaphragm.This new book presents topical research in the study of the types, symptoms and treatment of hernias.Topics discussed include minimally invasive repair of inguinal hernia in children; surgical approach to parastomal hernia and risk factors for incisional hernia after severe secondary peritonitis.

Chapter 1 - Inguinal hernia is the most common congenital defect for which pediatric surgeons perform surgery in daily practice. The principle of inguinal hernia repair in children is high ligation of the hernia sac.Open inguinal approaches have been the gold standard for childhood inguinal hernia repair. In the last decade, techniques of laparoscopy-assisted inguinal hernia repairs have been devised, and it has been shown that these methods are minimally invasive and produce satisfactory cosmetic results.These include intracorporeal suturing, the flip-flap technique, and extracorporeal knotting such as laparoscopic percutaneous extracorporeal closure (LPEC) and subcutaneous endoscopically assisted ligation (SEAL). Laparoscopy-assisted repairs offer a marked advantage in allowing contralateral exploration of a patent processus vaginalis (PPV) that may manifest as contralateral inguinal hernia later in life. However, there are technical problems in laparoscopy-assisted inguinal hernia repairs that include possible injuries to the vas and gonadal vessels, hydrocele formation, and a high incidence of hernia recurrence. The use of laparoscopy itself is sometimes disadvantageous due to laparoscopy-related complications. In addition, even if the laparoscopy is technically safe, routine exploration of a contralateral PPV and hernia repair in all patients with positive PPV has been criticized as overtreatment because the incidence of the positive PPV is much higher than the actual incidence of metachronous manifestation of contralateral inguinal hernia. Recently, another minimally invasive procedure for inguinal hernia repair in children, the selective sac extraction method (SSEM), was devised. SSEM is an innovative technique in which only the hernia sac is selectively extracted from the wound instead of elevating the entire cord structure. In female patients, the round ligament is elevated without pulling the surrounding muscular and fascial tissues out of the wound, resulting in hernia repair through an extremely minimal skin incision without performing laparoscopy. In this chapter, the history of the establishment of a simple high ligation as a method of inguinal hernia repair in children is reviewed. Following this, the advent of diagnostic and therapeutic laparoscopy and the development of minimally invasive procedures are reviewed, and an overview of the technical aspects of both laparoscopy-assisted repairs and SSEM is presented. Issues regarding contralateral exploration of PPV and surgical complications with inguinal hernia repairs in children are also discussed.

Chapter 2 - Parastomal hernia is an incisional abdominal wall hernia that involves a stoma. It is a common problem in patients with an intestinal stoma with an incidence of up to 50% or more.

Patients with stomas are at the highest risk of herniation during the initial 3-5 years after surgery, although hernia occurrence has been reported as late as 20 years after stoma creation. Herniation usually develops lateral to the stoma site.

Once a parastomal hernia has been diagnosed, seventy percent of the patients will be asymptomatic and can be managed nonoperatively. Typical reasons for surgical intervention include bowel obstruction, bowel strangulation, bleeding, pain, and poor fit of the stoma appliance.

Surgical therapy includes direct tissue repair of the defect, stoma relocation, and placement of a prosthetic mesh. Irrespective of technique, open repair is associated with high morbidity and non-mesh repair carries a high recurrence rate.

For local tissue repair of parastomal hernias and stoma relocation, recurrence is seen in 46 to 100% and 76% respectively. When utilizing prosthetics, a keyhole mesh configuration and, nonslit mesh repairs have been described. Dr Sugarbaker first described the nonslit mesh repair in 1980; this technique has been most effective, with the lowest recurrence rate.

The success of the Sugarbaker repair is attributed to the flap-valve action of the mesh on the bowel as it exits the peritoneal cavity and enters the abdominal wall. Minimally invasive approaches to parastomal hernia repair have gained popularity.

Mancini et al. described their experience with a laparoscopic modified Sugarbaker technique; patients were followed for 19 months and had a recurrence rate of 4%.

A review of literature supports the use of minimally invasive approach with prosthetic reinforcement as the optimal means of parastomal hernia repair.

Chapter 3 - The Greek term 'hernois' meaning bulge to describe abdominal hernias. The definition of hernia is 'A protrusion of any viscus from its proper cavity. There are abdominal, diaphragmatic, femoral, perineal, lumbar hernia ect. (classified according to the sites).Recognition of the typical appearance of various types of hernia and associated adverse features such as bowel obstruction, strangulation, incarceration, perforation or volvulus formation can help in formulating an accurate diagnosis. It is important to be familiar to hernia for all physicians because it can occur with morbidity and mortality. Thus, early and accurate diagnosis is important.

Chapter 4 - Introduction: Congenital diaphragmatic hernia (CDH) requiring a patch repair is likely to develop a more severe gastroesophageal reflux (GER) needing fundoplication during the first months of life. The author's hypothesis asserts that a prophylactic fundoplication performed during initial diaphragmatic repair can limit nutritional morbidity. The aim of this retrospective multicenter study was to clarify the relationship between prophylactic fundoplication and survival without growth disorder. Patients and methods: Between 1994 and 2005, 57 cases of left-side congenital diaphragmatic hernia requiring a patch repair were treated in 8 French pediatric surgery units. Prophylactic fundoplication was performed in 34 cases during initial diaphragmatic repair. Forty-three patients survived. Weight-for-height (W/H) and height-for-age (H/A) Z-scores were compared at 3 months, 3 and 5 years between the prophylactic fundoplication group (n=29) and the control group (n=14). The propensity score method was used to limit bias to determine if prophylactic fundoplication was an independent factor of survival without growth disorder (growth disorder was defined by weight-for-height and height-for-age Z-scores <-1.5 SD). Median follow-up was 4,88 years. Results: At 3 and 5 years, H/A Z-scores were significantly higher in prophylactic fundoplication group, -0.35 SD versus -1.19 SD (p=0.02) and -0.26 SD versus -1.31 SD (p=0.002). W/H Z-scores were not statistically different, -1.24 SD versus -1.62 SD (p>0.05) and -1.13 versus -1.4 SD (p>0.05). There was no significant difference between H/A and W/H Z-scores at 3 months or the need and the duration of gastric-tube feeding in the 2 groups. After adjustment for the propensity score, prophylactic fundoplication was significantly associated with survival without growth disorder (p=0.002). Conclusion: In this multicenter study concerning a high-risk population of congenital diaphragmatic hernia requiring a patch repair, there is a significant relationship between prophylactic fundoplication and survival without growth disorder after adjustment for the propensity score, suggesting that prophylactic fundoplication could prevents growth disorder. Furthermore, it was very interesting to note that prophylactic fundoplication only improved statural growth in these patients. These results must be confirmed by a prospective randomized study and a more detailed growth evaluation would be necessary to explain their unusual growth favouring height over weight.

Chapter 5 - The purpose of this chapter is to comprehensively review hiatal hernias, with particular attention paid to their pathophysiology and available treatment strategies. In this chapter, the Authors will dedicate a section discussing the dominant theories regarding the pathogenesis of hiatal hernias at the molecular and cellular level.

In addition, the Authors will review the surgical treatment strategies and their indications, with a particular emphasis on the indications for surgery which have changed drastically in recent years. Overall, there are two basic types of hiatal hernias, sliding and paraesophageal, each with a wide array of symptoms ranging from benign or asymptomatic to severe and fatal.

The most common symptoms observed are gastroesophageal reflux and dysphasia, and the treatment strategies employed are in large part to reduce the effects of these conditions while avoiding hernia recurrence.

Indeed, recent advancements in minimally invasive surgery have made the management of hiatal hernias radically different than a decade ago. Finally, the Authors will review the outcomes of surgical repairs including open, laparoscopic, and robotic approaches, and discuss the use of prosthetic meshes as an adjunct to the surgical treatment of this condition.

Chapter 6 - Laparoscopic surgery for pediatric inguinal hernia has been performed for over one-and-a-half decades. Numerous laparoscopic approaches have been reported, including intracorporeal ligation of the hernia defect with or without separation of the distal sac, and percutaneous endoscopically assisted ligation of the defect by variable devices.

However, there is no single laparoscopic approach that has fully replaced conventional inguinal herniotomy, since recurrence rate after laparoscopic surgery is generally known to be higher than after conventional inguinal herniotomy.

This chapter comprehensively reviews and compares the various laparoscopic techniques. There is a tendency toward diminishing the size and number of abdominal incisions and decreasing the usage of endoscopic instrumentation.

Single-port endoscopic-assisted percutaneous extraperitoneal closure seems to be the ultimate attainment. Technical evolution involving complete enclosure of the hernia defect without peritoneal gaps, the utility of preperitoneal hydrodissection, ligation of the defect with division of the distal sac, and double-ligation of the defect seems to be sufficient to achieve a low recurrence rate.

The future development of the technique is to move towards little invasiveness without complications, easy manipulation for widespread adoption, and recognition as a gold standard for the treatment of pediatric inguinal hernia.

Chapter 7 - *Background*: In patients with secondary peritonitis, infections of the abdominal cavity might render the abdominal wall susceptible to secondary complications like incisional hernia (IH). *Methods:* One hundred ninety-eight patients treated for secondary peritonitis underwent midline laparotomy.

Ninety-two surviving patients accessible to clinical follow-up were examined for the occurrence of IH and risk factors at the time of surgery or during follow-up were determined. *Results:* During a median follow-up period of 6 years 54.3% of the patients developed IHs.

A high body mass index, coronary heart disease, intense blood loss, requirement of intraoperative or postoperative transfusions and small bowel perforation as source of peritonitis were associated with IH. *Conclusion:* IH occurs quite frequently after surgery for secondary peritonitis.

Preexisting risk factors for IH and intraoperative blood loss or requirement of blood transfusions were correlated with the development of IH. Interestingly, surgical technique was not correlated with the development of IH in this series.

Chapter 8 - Congenital umbilical hernia is the most common abdominal wall defect in children. Most surgeons agree to pursue nonoperative management before age 5 unless the hernia is symptomatic, incarcerated or strangulated. Umbilical hernias in adults comprise only 6% of all abdominal wall hernias, with over 90% of these defects being acquired, presenting in the fifth or sixth decades of life. Etiologies are multifactorial. Typical adult umbilical hernia patients include: those with a history of prostatic hypertrophy, chronic obstructive pulmonary disease (COPD), constipation, hepatic cirrhosis with ascites, morbid obesity and multiparous women. The umbilical hernia sack may include omentum, small bowel and colon. Incarceration and strangulation of abdominal viscera in umbilical hernias is 14-fold more likely in adults than in children. Adult umbilical hernias rarely resolve spontaneously, and strong consideration should be given to prompt repair because of its association with increased morbidity and mortality. Traditionally, umbilical hernia repair is an open procedure, but recently several laparoscopic or laparoscopic-assisted approaches have been described. The use of mesh has drastically changed the surgical approach to hernia repair, demonstrating a dramatic decrease in hernia recurrence rates. But the use of mesh produces its own unique complications: rarely patients can present with bowel obstruction due to adhesions to the mesh, hernia recurrence can occur as a result of mesh contraction, and cases of complete mesh migration into small bowel have been reported. Postoperative pain is usually well controlled. Interestingly, when laparoscopic approach is used, fixation of mesh with transabdominal sutures is a unique source of prolonged postoperative pain. Following simple suture repair or Mayo repair, recurrence rates range from 11% to 54%. The use of mesh has lowered the recurrence rate to 1%. The lower recurrence rate with mesh is most likely a result of tension-free repair.

Chapter 9 - Eventration disease is the protrusion of abdominal contents through a defect in the abdominal wall. The hole represents more than an imperfection. It decouples the counterbalancing mechanical forces of the lateral abdominal musculature. This gradual change in abdominal wall mechanics leads to compensatory mechanisms that in turn lead to further herniation. The purpose of this chapter is to comprehensively review the relevant history, pathophysiology, and treatment strategies of ventral incisional hernias.

As there exists a large volume of inconsistent data on methodology of incisional herniorraphy, particular attention has been dedicated to clinical approaches described by evidence-based literature. Additionally, this work includes a detailed discussion of the theory, design, and application of implantable materials. Furthermore, the authors describe the evolution of autologous tissue abdominal wall reconstructive procedures and their evolving integration with minimally invasive technologies. Finally, a brief discussion is held outlining the current evidence that supports mesh fixation techniques.

Chapter 10 - A Spigelian hernia is a congenital or acquired defect in the spigelian aponeurosis of anterior abdominal wall. It is present in up to 2% of the population with hernia defects and is most commonly seen in the fourth to seventh decade of life. This aponeurosis is located between the semilunar line (laterally) and the lateral edge of the rectus muscle (medially). This defect is most commonly found in the spigelian belt which is a 6 cm area superior to a line between the anterior superior iliac spines and below the arcuate line. Greater omentum is usually seen incarcerated between the muscles of the lateral abdominal wall and is oftentimes difficult to appreciate on physical exam. These are usually smaller sized defects and thus the danger comes when the patient has an incarcerated or strangulated section of small or large bowel. Diagnosis of Spigelian hernias is via Computed Tomography scans, ultrasound or at the time of surgery for a small bowel obstruction or peritonitis. The key to diagnosis is clinical suspicion as well as a thorough history, physical exam and appropriate work-up. Surgical treatment has traditionally been performed through an open approach with a primary closure of the fascia or placement of mesh. More recently, surgeons have demonstrated that both the diagnosis and repair of these hernias can be accomplished laparoscopically with minimal morbidity. Both techniques reportedly have very low recurrence rates and patients with these hernias tend to do well.

In: Hernias: Types, Symptoms and Treatment
Editor: James H. Wagner

ISBN: 978-1-61324-125-7
© 2011 Nova Science Publishers, Inc.

Chapter 1

Minimally Invasive Repair of Inguinal Hernias in Children

Hiotshi Ikeda[*]
Department of Pediatric Surgery, Dokkyo Medical University Koshigaya Hospital, Koshigaya, Saitama, Japan

Introduction

Inguinal hernia is the most common congenital defect for which pediatric surgeons perform surgery in daily practice. The principle of inguinal hernia repair in children is high ligation of the hernia sac. Open inguinal approaches have been the gold standard for childhood inguinal hernia repair. In the last decade, techniques of laparoscopy-assisted inguinal hernia repairs have been devised, and it has been shown that these methods are minimally invasive and produce satisfactory cosmetic results. These include intracorporeal suturing, the flip-flap technique, and extracorporeal knotting such as laparoscopic percutaneous extracorporeal closure (LPEC) and subcutaneous endoscopically assisted ligation (SEAL). Laparoscopy-assisted repairs offer a marked advantage in allowing

---

[*]Tel: 048-965-1111, Fax: 048-965-8927, E-mail: hike@dokkyomed.ac.jp

contralateral exploration of a patent processus vaginalis (PPV) that may manifest as contralateral inguinal hernia later in life. However, there are technical problems in laparoscopy-assisted inguinal hernia repairs that include possible injuries to the vas and gonadal vessels, hydrocele formation, and a high incidence of hernia recurrence. The use of laparoscopy itself is sometimes disadvantageous due to laparoscopy-related complications. In addition, even if the laparoscopy is technically safe, routine exploration of a contralateral PPV and hernia repair in all patients with positive PPV has been criticized as overtreatment because the incidence of the positive PPV is much higher than the actual incidence of metachronous manifestation of contralateral inguinal hernia. Recently, another minimally invasive procedure for inguinal hernia repair in children, the selective sac extraction method (SSEM), was devised. SSEM is an innovative technique in which only the hernia sac is selectively extracted from the wound instead of elevating the entire cord structure. In female patients, the round ligament is elevated without pulling the surrounding muscular and fascial tissues out of the wound, resulting in hernia repair through an extremely minimal skin incision without performing laparoscopy. In this chapter, the history of the establishment of a simple high ligation as a method of inguinal hernia repair in children is reviewed. Following this, the advent of diagnostic and therapeutic laparoscopy and the development of minimally invasive procedures are reviewed, and an overview of the technical aspects of both laparoscopy-assisted repairs and SSEM is presented. Issues regarding contralateral exploration of PPV and surgical complications with inguinal hernia repairs in children are also discussed.

I. Inguinal Hernia Repair by Simple High Ligation: A Historical Review

After reviewing original articles in the late nineteenth century, it is clear that most children with inguinal hernia at that time were treated by a truss, and that the dominant opinion among surgeons regarding the treatment of childhood inguinal hernia was a time-honored doctrine. Hamilton R. Russell (Figure 1), a surgeon who was born in England and practiced surgery in Australia, criticized such a doctrine in his article in 1899 entitled "The etiology and treatment of inguinal hernia in the young."[1] It tells us how children of his age with inguinal hernia were treated, and the dissenting opinion of Dr. Russell was as follows:

"Operation for hernia should never be undertaken in the case of a young child when the hernia is susceptible of efficient control by a truss, for in a large number of cases treatment by truss for a time will result in cure of the rupture (hernia)."

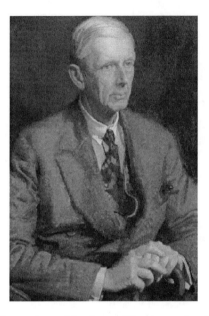

Figure 1. Portrait of Hamilton R. Russell by George Washington Lambert, a painter in the 1920s (From Royle JP. College portraits, surgeons and the Archibald Prize. ANZ J Surg 2005; 75:483-488. Copyright John Wiley and Sons).

This meant that surgery was used only in the most serious cases in which truss treatment was inefficient or incarceration had occurred. Banks mentioned in his article published in 1882 that he had a strong belief that a well-fitting truss worn constantly to the age of fifteen would cure the great majority of hernias in children under ten years of age [2]. Surprisingly, it was also reported that almost 1,200 deaths occurred annually from strangulated hernia in the UK, although it was unknown whether strangulation developed as a result of inefficient truss treatment. Against the opinions of the majority of surgeons, Russell insisted that truss treatment was much more uncertain and inefficient than was generally supposed and that it should be discredited and abondoned[1].

Russell clearly stated that inguinal hernia in children was due to the presence of a congenital sac, patent processus vaginalis, and that the removal of the sac in early life could completely cure the hernia. He was the first surgeon who suggested that simple high ligation of the sac was sufficient to cure inguinal hernia in children. His theory on the etiology and treatment of childhood inguinal hernia led him into conflict with the authorities of his time, but Russell's idea proved to be valid and was finally endorsed by his British and American colleagues. The practice of simple high ligation alone became the principle repair for inguinal hernia in children that is still employed by modern pediatric surgeons. In Russell's operation, the main procedure was ligation and removal of the hernia sac at its neck after separation from the cord. In his operation, the testes were drawn out of the scrotum, which is no longer performed in modern repairs. Russell's operation was described in his article as follows[1]:

> "The incision is made in the groin, parallel to Poupart's (inguinal) ligament, the cord is sought for, the coverings of the cord are successively opened, and the cord, the sac, and the testicle are drawn out of the scrotum. The vas deferens and the vessels of the cord are next defined and separated from the sac and the sac is freed from these structures as high up in the canal as possible. A chromicised catgut ligature is now applied to the neck of the sac in the form of the Staffordshire knot and the sac is removed, the superfluous coverings of the cord are cut away, and the testicle is carefully washed and dried and replaced in the scrotum. The wound in the groin is closed by the subcuticular method of suturing, a single thread of silkworm gut being used for this purpose, the two ends of which emerge from the skin about half an inch from either extremity of the wound."

It took more than half a century for surgery to become the standard treatment of inguinal hernia in children. Willis J. Potts of Chicago mentioned in his original paper published in 1950 that innumerable articles had advised prolonged truss treatment, delaying the operation until the child was two to four years old, and all sorts of complicated methods of plastic repair of the muscles and fascial structures[3]. In the late nineteenth century, there were two different principles of repair in inguinal hernia in adults. One was a reinforcement of the anterior wall of the inguinal canal and a tightening of the external inguinal ring, and the other was a reinforcement of the posterior wall of the inguinal canal and a tightening of the internal inguinal ring[4]. In 1877, a German surgeon, Vinzenz von Czerny, reported surgical reinforcement of external oblique muscle aponeurosis by fascial duplication without opening the aponeurosis. This was performed to narrow the external inguinal ring, but the recurrence rate was unfortunately high with this type of anterior plasty of the inguinal canal, which led to the innovation of methods for posterior reinforcement of the inguinal canal. In 1881, a French surgeon, Just Lucas-Championnière, pointed out that a ligature of the hernia sac high up on the internal inguinal ring should be performed after splitting the external oblique aponeurosis. Then, in 1889 an Italian surgeon, Eduardo Bassini, published a text on operative methods of inguinal hernia, in which he described a method of posterior reinforcement of the inguinal canal by fastening a threefold layer of the internal oblique muscle, the transverse abdominal muscle, and the transversalis fascia to the posterior edge of the inguinal ligament[4]. Thereafter, posterior reinforcement was the standard of inguinal hernia surgery, and it was applied not only to repairs in adults, but also to those in children, until Potts emphasized that the cause of indirect inguinal hernia in children was not muscular weakness, but failure of the processus vaginalis to obliterate. He concluded that surgical treatment should consist of a simple removal of the offending sac and nothing more, and that high ligation of the sac alone would suffice to cure inguinal hernia in children.

Potts also mentioned that the problem of hernia in children was often dismissed with a few sentences, or the principles governing treatment in adults were inappropriately applied to children[3]. A kind of indifference or ignorance may have been present despite the fact that Russell had published an article on his pioneering work more than 50 years earlier. After Russell's work, several surgeons repeatedly suggested that mere simple high ligation or removal of the sac, rather than plastic repairs of the inguinal canal, would suffice to cure inguinal hernia in children. Potts listed the surgeons who had contributed to form the principle of treatment of inguinal hernia in children. Turner in 1912 advised complete removal of the sac at the internal inguinal ring through a small incision made on the aponeurosis of the external oblique muscle[5]. He added that any attempt to strengthen the inguinal canal was unnecessary. In 1924, Russell addressed his operative procedure of inguinal hernia at the King's Medical Society in New York and re-emphasized that a mere removal of the sac was sufficient for repair of oblique (inguinal) hernia in children, a speech that was published the following year[6]. Herzfeld presented an experience of an operative method performed in an outpatient clinic, by which the sac was ligated through the external inguinal ring, in 1938[7]. The procedure was quite similar to one originally presented by Banks, and he partially closed the external inguinal ring as Banks did[2]. Coles in 1945, supporting Turner's approach, advised transection of the sac, of which the proximal part was transfixed and highly ligated, while the distal part of the sac was left without further treatment[8].

He also stressed that extensive dissection of the sac with plastic repair of the inguinal canal should be abandoned because inguinal hernia in children was not due to any weakness of the inguinal structures, but solely to the presence of a processus vaginalis. Coles disapproved of Herzfeld's procedures that were performed by many European surgeons of his age, explaining that pulling the neck of the sac down through the external inguinal ring without opening the inguinal canal was not a safe procedure. Coles' operation was basically the same as Potts' operation described below.

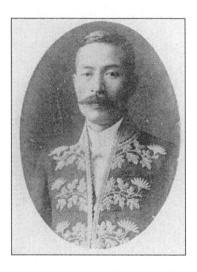

Figure 2. Portrait of Toyoo Yatsushiro (Courtesy of Professor Shizu Sakai, Department of Medical History, Juntendo University).

In the Far East, a Japanese surgeon, Toyoo Yatsushiro (Figure 2), probably after learning from surgical authorities on the other side of the globe, believed that high ligation and transection should be performed as soon as possible when inguinal hernia was diagnosed and that plastic repairs of the inguinal canal were rather injurious in children. These points were mentioned in his article published in 1911[9]. Potts' operation, the principles of which were not originally his idea, became the standard procedure for inguinal hernia in children. The procedure has been performed by many pediatric surgeons who followed Potts, although with minor modifications. The original description of Potts' operation was as follows (Figure 3)[3]:

> "In all infants below approximately two years of age a one inch transverse skin incision is made in the crease which crosses the baby's abdomen in the suprapubic region. Such a skin incision is easier to close and less apt to become infected than an oblique incision, and because it follows the lines of cleavage it heals more smoothly with a scarcely visible scar and without

annoying keloid formation. Cosmetic reasons for a minimal scar in the inguinal region carry little weight with the surgeon but are a source of pride to the mother. Why make an ugly scar anywhere when a neat one is possible with no more effort? In older children likewise, a transverse incision rather than one parallel with Poupart's ligament is made in the proper location."

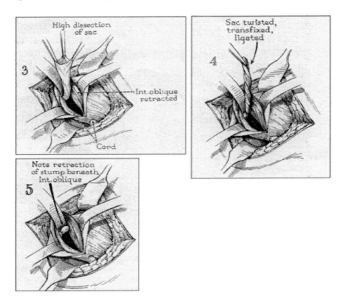

Figure 3. Parts of the original figure of Potts' operation (From Potts WJ, et al. The treatment of inguinal hernia in infants and children. Ann Surg 1950; 132:566-576. Copyright Wolters Kluwer Health).

In modern pediatric surgery, compared to the dawn of pediatric surgery, cosmesis is of much more concern and the appearance of incisional scars are more important factors when any surgical methods are considered. Infants and children who undergo surgery have to grow up and live for several decades or more with scars. Potts was concerned about incisional scars, and in all likelihood, he was probably the first pediatric surgeon who described cosmetic reasons for his selection of skin incision:

"The external oblique is opened parallel with its fibers, but in routine cases the external ring is not opened. The lower half of the external oblique is retracted downward, while with a Halsted clamp the cremasteric fibers are split parallel with the cord, and the sac, easily recognizable by its gray-white color, is grasped and lifted up. With great gentleness the vessels and vas are dissected from the fragile sac as far upward as possible. The sac in infants is often as thin as gossamer and must be handled very gently or it will tear and become difficult to identify and to close properly. The interior of the sac is inspected for the presence of intestine or omentum and in female for ovary or tube. The sac is then twisted until the properitoneal fat appears or until the neck of the sac has been completely obliterated. The sac is then transfixed high with a silk suture and tied snugly. The excess is cut away. Attempts at transfixion and ligation of the neck of the sac without twisting will often lead to tearing and improper closure. The external oblique fibers are coapted with a few interrupted fine silk sutures. The superficial fascia and subcutaneous fat are apposed and the skin is closed."

Potts' operation became a standard procedure that is still used in modern repair of inguinal hernia in children. Since it is the shortest way to the internal inguinal ring and the base of the sac, the inguinal canal is opened by an incision in the aponeurosis of the external oblique muscle instead of entering the canal from the external inguinal ring.

When open surgery is necessary for incarceration, the aponeurosis of the external oblique muscle is usually incised from the external inguinal ring. Potts also clearly mentioned where the sac should be transfixed and ligated. It is necessary to confirm the preperitoneal (expressed as "properitoneal" in Potts' original article) fat tissue before ligation.

Variations in Procedure

Mitchell Banks' Operation

The majority of surgeons in modern pediatric practice approach the inguinal canal through an incision in the external oblique muscle aponeurosis. In young infants, the internal inguinal ring is so close to the external ring that the hernia sac and cord structures can be approached without opening the external oblique aponeurosis. This alternative to approaching the sac was performed by surgeons including Herzfeld[7] and Kurlan [10], and is known as the Mitchell Banks technique. The procedure was described as follows[10]:

"The spermatic cord or the round ligament is isolated at the level at the external inguinal ring. Then the hernia sac, usually lying on the anteromedial aspect, is dissected free from the margins of the external ring and isolated from the spermatic cord or round ligament, where it is doubly ligated with fine 3-0 or 4-0 silk sutures and excised. If the external ring is enlarged, the medial and lateral pillars are coapted with two or three 4-0 chromic catgut sutures."

Since the inguinal canal is quite short in infants, the internal and external inguinal rings lie in proximity. In such cases, the sac can be identified, dissected from the cord structures, and adequately ligated as high as possible from the external inguinal ring.

Although quite rare in children, when the posterior wall is weakened, additional plasty for the inguinal canal is difficult with this approach[11]. Actually, Banks himself applied this procedure to repairs in adult patients and only one of his patients was a young infant[2]. Herzfeld was one of the surgeons who advocated Banks' procedure in hernia repair in children.[7]

Marcy's Operation

Griffith stated, in his chapter on Marcy's operation, that the principle of high ligation alone in all hernia repairs in children does not always suffice. Supporting the principle concepts of Marcy's operation, he wrote the following[12]:

"High ligation alone applies only when the sac is found to have a tiny neck that does not even admit a fingertip. In these infants and children the internal ring is obviously not enlarged and therefore does not require repair, but many children, and some infants also, have sacs with patulous necks that readily admit a finger or even a thumb into the peritoneal cavity. These patulous necks signify that the internal ring is also patulous. Fascial repair of the internal ring is therefore performed with one or more sutures. This repair is done to prevent indirect recurrence, which in many instances does not appear until adulthood."

Marcy's operation for inguinal hernia consists of removing the sac and repairing the internal inguinal ring by closing the defect or hole in the transversalis fascia. It was indicated that closure of the internal inguinal ring completed the Marcy operation and there was nothing to be added in children[12]. Such a plasty of the posterior wall of the inguinal canal, however, is usually unnecessary in repairs in children.

II. The Era of Laparoscopic Repairs

Diagnostic Laparoscopy and Contralateral Exploration

Laparoscopy was initially introduced more as a diagnostic tool than as a therapeutic approach in groin hernias. It provides intracorporeal visualization of the inguinal region from the inside and can give an accurate diagnosis of non-indirect inguinal hernias, as well as indirect inguinal hernias.

Direct inguinal hernia and femoral hernia are relatively uncommon in children, and a diagnosis of direct hernia based solely on physical findings is usually difficult. Although direct hernia has been assumed to be extremely rare in children, laparoscopic examination revealed that it was found in 0.5%-2.6% of children with groin hernias[13-16].

Femoral hernia were also found in 1%-2.6% of children with a bulge in the groin, and these patients are sometimes misdiagnosed as having inguinal hernia[14,15]. This data indicates that laparoscopy is a useful way of making a correct diagnosis of groin hernias.

Contralateral Exploration

Diagnostic laparoscopy is used more often in contralateral exploration than in only making accurate diagnoses of hernia (Figure 4). The presence of a PPV on the contralateral side can be explored by laparoscopy when unilateral inguinal hernia is repaired. When the contralateral side is positive for PPV, it can be treated at the same time as the ipsilateral hernia repair is implemented.

The indication for contralateral exploration, however, has been controversial regarding surgery in children with inguinal hernia since the 1950s, when several investigators reported a high incidence of PPV on the contralateral side[17,18]. Discussions regarding routine bilateral exploration can be summarized as follows[18]: the advantages of the procedure include the avoidance of a second operation, anesthesia, and a reduction in overall cost, whereas the disadvantages include overtreatment due to otherwise unnecessary operations and the possibility of complications. The reported incidence of metachronous contralateral inguinal hernia is 5.8% to 11.6%[19-26].

The risk of contralateral manifestation is high in patients with left-side hernia and patients with a family history (accumulation of inguinal hernia in family members within the second degree relationship) (Table 1)[24]. The incidence is 10% to 13% in these high-risk patients [24-27], but is still much lower than the incidence of PPV, at 48% to 61%[18,28,29]. Since a positive PPV does not necessarily cause clinical manifestations of inguinal hernia, surgical intervention for every PPV has been criticized as overtreatment.

At the same time, such intervention may cause complications including damage to the vas deferens and testicular vessels, testicular atrophy, and testicular dislocation[20]. On the other hand, closure of a PPV effectively reduces the incidence of metachronous contralateral hernia. Only a small number of patients returned with a hernia after a negative exploration by means of either a diagnostic pneumoperitoneum test, the Goldstein test, or laparoscopy[30-33].

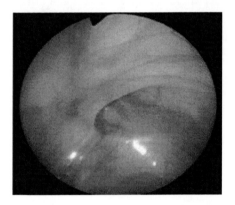

Figure 4. Laparoscopic view of a patent processus vaginalis in a female patient.

Table 1 Risk of contralateral manifestation in patients with unilateral inguinal hernia

Characteristics	Hazard ratio (95% CI)	p value
Left side hernia	1.40 (1.02-1.90)	0.037
Age at repair		
< 6 mo	1.21 (0.85-1.73)	0.292
< 12 mo	1.18 (0.86-1.61)	0.319
Family history of inguinal hernia	1.59 (1.10-2.29)	0.013

(Reprinted from J Pediatr Surg, Ikeda H, et al., Risk of contralateral manifestation in children with unilateral inguinal hernia: should hernia in children be treated contralaterally? 2000; 35:1746-1748, with permission from Elsevier)

Contralateral exploration can be accomplished either by a port placed at an umbilical incision (umbilical approach) or a trocar placed through the ipsilateral hernia sac (transinguinal approach)[34]. In particular, the latter approach was introduced into clinical practice in the 1990s[32,33,35]. It provides excellent evaluation of the internal inguinal ring contralaterally by using angled (30-degrees to 120-degrees) endoscopes[36,37]. The criteria for positive PPV is the presence of a significant peritoneal opening at the internal inguinal ring, the absence of an identifiable termination of the peritoneal sac, or the expression of bubbles by palpating the inguinal canal[37]. Laparoscopy, regardless of an umbilical or transinguinal approach, offers a safe and effective means to confirm the presence of PPV during ipsilateral hernia repair. No high-level evidence has been presented to conclude whether a relatively high incidence of PPV and low incidence of the metachronous manifestation of hernia justify routine contralateral exploration. However, most pediatric surgeons who practice laparoscopic repairs perform simultaneous explorations by laparoscopy [24,38,39]. Whether performing contralateral exploration or not is usually dependent on the parents' preference, so the decision should be made on an informed consent basis. Since the method certainly benefits patients in whom second surgery and anesthesia have to be avoided due to complications such as respiratory or cardiovascular problems, it should be reserved particularly for these high-risk children [24].

Laparoscopic Repairs of Inguinal Hernia in Children

Simple high ligation of the hernia sac by an open inguinal approach has been a standard procedure worldwide and has been used widely for inguinal hernia repair in children. However, the introduction of diagnostic laparoscopy has led to the advent of therapeutic laparoscopy in children with inguinal hernia, as well as adults. A number of articles on innovative laparoscopic repairs have been published. In1997, El-Gohary first reported an experience of laparoscopic ligation of the hernia sac in female patients[40]. He inverted the hernia sac and ligated its base by applying endoscopic loops under laparoscopic visualization. A total of 28 patients were treated by the method with only one recurrence reported. The original description of the method is as follows:

> "The diagnosis was confirmed using a 5-mm telescope induced via a supraumbilical incision. Two 5-mm ports were introduced, one into each flank. An endoscopic loop was then introduced from the side contralateral to

the hernia to be ligated. A grasper was introduced via the ipsilateral port into the internal ring. The hernial sac was grasped at a point as far as possible from the internal ring and inverted through the loop into the abdominal cavity. The loop was then secured around the base of the sac."

After El-Gohary's method was presented, technical innovations and modifications have been reported one after another, extending the techniques to male patients. These methods can be divided into two categories based on the approach used to close the hernia sac. These are intraperitoneal and extraperitoneal approaches[41].

Intraperitoneal Approaches

This category includes El-Gohary's method (endolooping), suturing of the internal inguinal ring, the flip-flap technique, and their modifications. In 1998, Schier reported intraabdominal suturing of the open internal rings with Z-sutures of a non-absorbable material [42]. He modified his techniques and tried purse-string or N-shaped sutures of a 4-0 monofilament suture, and reported the results of 712 repairs in 542 children [13,14]. According to the report, there were 4.1% hernia recurrences, 0.7% hydroceles, and 0.2% testicular atrophies, while wound cosmesis was excellent. He mentioned that all recurrences occurred between the suture and the epigastric vessels and believed that sutures had been placed too far laterally out of fear of injuring the vas and epigastric vessels[14]. He also reported that direct hernias were found in 2.3%-2.6% of cases. Since direct hernia have been regarded as uncommon in children, it is often excluded from the preoperative differential diagnosis of groin hernias. It is sometimes diagnosed only after high ligation of the processus vaginalis fails to resolve a bulge in the groin. Direct hernia may not be as uncommon as generally believed, as previously mentioned (see the section on diagnostic laparoscopy).

Montupet et al. reported a similar experience of inguinal hernia repair using a purse-string suture of a 3-0 absorbable suture[43]. He cut the periorificial peritoneum laterally to the internal inguinal ring to facilitate suture and closure of the hernia sac. An approximation of the conjoined tendon and the crural arch using sutures with a nonabsorbable suture was added. A total of 47 inguinal hernias in 45 boys were repaired and 2 (4.4%) experienced hernia recurrence.

Shalaby et al. closed the internal inguinal ring by a technique using a Reverdin needle under a needlescope[44]. The two ends of the thread were passed through the margins of the ring, withdrawn through the port, and tied by an extracorporeal knot. No recurrence or hydrocele formation was reported.

The flip-flap technique, reported by Yip et al. in 2004, is a unique method of inguinal hernia repair via an intraperitoneal approach in which the internal inguinal ring is not tightly ligated and a peritoneal flap anchored with a nonabsorbable suture closes the hernia opening in a tension-free manner [45]. The technique was used in 43 inguinal hernia repairs and no recurrence was observed over a relatively short follow-up period. The idea of the flip-flap and the preliminary results of the original report were appealing, but the results of the subsequent study were unfortunately very poor[46]. Of the 15 patients who underwent hernia repair using the laparoscopic flip-flap technique, the vas deferens was injured in one patient and the flaps were torn during suturing in 3 patients. Hernia recurrence was observed in 4 patients up to 3 months postoperatively, which led to the conclusion that until more studies to verify the usefulness of the method were done, it could not be justified.

Another laparoscopic repair without ligation of the hernia sac was presented by Riquelme et al[47]. He resected the hernia sac and the parietal peritoneum surrounding the internal inguinal ring, anticipating that peritoneal scarring would seal the inguinal canal and close the internal inguinal ring. A purse-string suture was used when the internal ring was wider than 10 mm. The method was performed in 91 patients and no recurrence was observed during the follow-up of up to 4 years.

Giseke et al. also reported laparoscopic herniotomy, which consisted of a circumferential incision of the peritoneum around the hernia sac at the internal inguinal ring and a closure of the peritoneum by suture with a nonabsorbable suture[15]. The recurrence rate was 1% among 385 children. The results were fascinating and promising, but well-trained laparoscopic surgeons were indispensable to accomplish intraperitoneal resection of the hernia sac.

Extraperitoneal Approaches

In 2001, Endo et al. reported laparoscopic extraperitoneal ligation of the hernia sac with a 2-0 nonabsorbable twine using a specially designed Endoneedle for sending and retrieving a suture (Figure 5)[48]. The method was applied in more than 1,200 patients, showing excellent results with 0.2% incidence of hernia recurrence[49]. After Endo described his original method, various minor modifications of the technique or the use of innovative instruments have been reported. These reports unequivocally stress that laparoscopic repair by extraperitoneal ligation of the hernia sac is safe and minimally invasive, and that cosmetic results are excellent. The incidence of hernia recurrence was not significantly variable among the reports.

Lee et al. performed high purse-string ligation extraperitoneally with a microlaparoscope using innovative instruments in 450 patients, which resulted in small incisions, a short operation time, and a quick recovery from surgery[50]. Hernia recurrence was observed in 4 patients (0.88%) after 6 to 18 months of follow-up.

Harrison et al. used a swaged needle which was guided extraperitoneally around the internal inguinal ring by a Touhy needle, and devised the see-saw maneuver to avoid injury to the vas and spermatic vessels (Figure 6)[51]. The method was dubbed subcutaneous endoscopically assisted ligation (SEAL), and was applied to 300 repairs of inguinal hernia in children[52]. Absorbable sutures were used in 40% of repairs and nonabsorbable sutures in the remainder. There were 13 (4.3%) hernia recurrences and 7 hydrocele formations. Of the 13 cases of hernia recurrence, 6 underwent SEAL with absorbable sutures and 7 with nonabsorbable sutures. The avarage time from SEAL to hernia recurrence was 3.3 months. In Harrison's method, using a swaged needle with a Touhy needle is difficult under two-dimensional visualization.

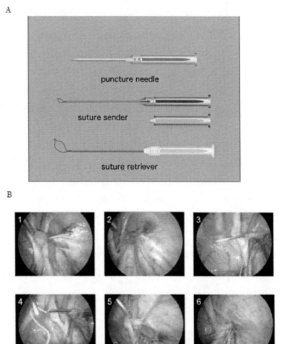

Figure 5. Instruments and laparoscopic views of the Endo's method. (A) Specially designed Endoneedles for sending and retrieving a suture. (B) The hernia sac is ligated extraperitoneally with a 2-0 nonabsorbable twine (Courtesy of Masao Endo, M.D., Ex-director, Department of Pediatric Surgery, Saitama City Hospital, Saitama, Japan).

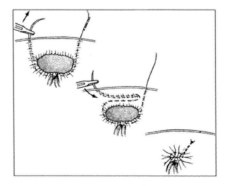

Figure 6. A swaged-on needle is backed through the subcutaneous tissue by the see-saw maneuver. Under direct endoscopic observation, the patent processus is closed at the internal ring (Reprinted from J Pediatr Surg, Harrison MR, et al. Subcutaneous endoscopically assisted ligation (SEAL) of the internal ring for repair of inguinal hernias in children: A novel technique. J Pediatr Surg 2005; 40:1177-1180, with permission from Elsevier).

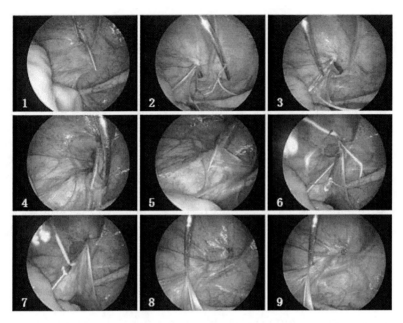

Figure 7. Laparoscopic views of the LPEC procedure (Courtesy of Hiroo Takehara, M.D., Director, Department of Pediatric Surgery and Pediatric Endosurgery, Tokushima University Hospital, Tokushima, Japan).

Laparoscopic percutaneous extraperitoneal closure (LPEC), reported by Takehara et al. in 2006, was another modification (Figure 7)[16]. A special needle with a wire loop was used to place a suture circumferentially around the internal inguinal ring. The method was performed in 972 repairs, 40 of which were accomplished with a 3-0 absorbable suture, while the rest were done with a 2-0 nonabsorbable suture. A retrospective analysis showed that there were 6 (0.73%) recurrences, 5 of which were among the repairs with absorbable sutures. Direct hernia, whose diagnosis is usually difficult even after opening the inguinal canal in children, was laparoscopically diagnosed in 7 (0.98%) patients. The patients were treated laparoscopically by LPEC with an additional iliopubic tract repair. Double extraperitoneal ligation of the internal inguinal ring with nonabsorbable sutures placed by a hernia hook were performed in 577 hernia repairs, and the recurrence rate was 0.35%[53].

Technical Problems in Laparoscopic Repairs

Pediatric surgeons who advocate laparoscopic repairs stress that their methods are safe and minimally invasive, and that surgery results in less pain, an earlier postoperative recovery, and more satisfactory wound cosmesis compared to conventional open surgeries[54]. However, there are technical problems, including possible injuries to the vas and testicular vessels, hydrocele formation, and a relatively high incidence of hernia recurrence. Because the vas and testicular vessels are just beneath the peritoneum of the posterior hemicircumference of the internal inguinal ring, the needle can injure these vital structures in male patients regardless of an intraperitoneal or extraperitoneal approach. Suture or ligation to close the hernia sac may cause irreversible injuries to the vas and testicular vessels, which are sometimes invisible under a laparoscope. Saline injection into the extraperitoneal space can lift the peritoneum and may effectively keep these structures away from sutures or ligation.

Hernia Recurrence after Laparoscopic Repairs

The incidence of postoperative hernia recurrence seems to be higher in laparoscopic repairs compared to conventional open repairs (Table 2). In particular, the incidence is seemingly higher when repaired by intraperitoneal approaches than by extraperitoneal approaches. In conventional open repairs, recurrence is thought to be caused by several factors. Failure to identify the hernia sac during the original procedure inevitably results in the reappearance of a bulge in the groin soon after surgery. Failure to ligate the sac highly enough at the internal ring or a tear in the sac by which a strip of peritoneum remains along the cord structures are also assumed to be reasons for postoperative recurrence[55]. Damage to the floor of the inguinal canal during the original procedure may cause postoperative direct hernia. If a direct hernia is missed at the original procedure, symptoms remain postoperatively. As for laparoscopic repairs, several technical refinements have been proposed to reduce the incidence of recurrence. Chan et al. showed that tensionless repair could prevent hernia recurrence in repairs by intraperitoneal approaches[56]. The incidence decreased from 4.88% to 0.4% after adoption of technical routines including an extraperitoneal saline injection to reduce the size of the internal inguinal ring, confirmation of knot airtightness, and an addition of a second purse-string stitch when needed. By observing the inguinal region laparoscopically in recurrent hernias, Treef and Schier revealed that most recurrences occurred medially to the previous suture and that the knot had become loose in some cases [57]. They suggested that the stitches at the medial side of the hernia in the vicinity of the vas were crucial, and believed that the more experienced the surgeon, the fewer incidences of recurrence.

Table 2. Laparoscopic repairs and hernia recurrence in children with inguinal hernia

Repair (approach and method)	Author	Hernia recurrence (%)
I Intraperitoneal approaches		
Endoloop	El-Gohary[40]	3.6
Suture		
Purse-string, Z-shaped, N-shaped	Schier[13,14]	3.4-4.1
Purse-string	Montupet[43]	4.4
Reverdin needle	Shalaby[44]	0
Flip-flap	Yip[45]	0
	Hassan[46]	27
Resection of the sac	Riquelme[47]	0
Resection and suture	Giseke[15]	1
II Extraperitoneal approaches		
Ligation	Endo[49]	0.2
	Lee[50]	0.88
	Ozgediz[52]	4.3
	Takehara[16]	0.73
	Tam[53]	0.35

Another study performed by Marte et al. suggested that the addition of an incision laterally to the intraperitoneal suture of the internal inguinal ring may effectively prevent hernia recurrence due to better sealing of the ring [58].

What Are the Benefits of Laparoscopic Repairs?

It is believed, as described above, that laparoscopic repairs are associated with less pain, a smoother postoperative recovery, and more satisfactory wound cosmesis compared to conventional open repairs[41]. However, recent studies suggested that while laparoscopic repairs are clearly superior procedures in terms of cosmesis and can detect contralateral PPV, recoveries and outcomes are similar for both laparoscopic and open repairs[59-61]. The advantages of laparoscopic repairs include clear visualization of the internal inguinal ring from the inside, easy assessment of the processus vaginalis contralateral patency, easy inspection of abdominal and pelvic viscera, and particular wound cosmesis. The disadvantages include the need for endotracheal intubation and the potential risks of injury to intraabdominal organs from laparoscopy, trocars, and other instruments. When laparoscopic and conventional open repairs are compared, the best clinical treatment is not yet clear [62,63].

III. Minimally Invasive Hernia Repair Without Laparoscopy: A Selective Sac Extraction Method (SSEM)

In 2009, Ikeda et al. reported a novel technique for inguinal hernia repair in children [64]. It was devised to achieve satisfactory surgical and cosmetic results with minimal surgical invasiveness without laparoscopic assistance. It was dubbed the selective sac extraction method (SSEM). In SSEM, the hernia sac is selectively extracted and highly ligated through an extremely small skin incision.

SSEM Procedure in Male Patients (Figure 8)

Because the skin incision of the SSEM is very small, approximately 5 mm in length, it has to be located at the skin just above the internal inguinal ring. In children with inguinal hernia, the spermatic cord structure is easily located by palpation. It is thickened and feels as if two pieces of silky cloth are being rubbed. A small skin crease incision is made where the spermatic cord overlies the pectineal line of the pubic bone lateral to the pubic tubercle. Then, the two superficial fascias, Camper's and Scarpa's fascias, are grasped, elevated with small mosquito clamps, and incised. The aponeurosis of the external oblique muscle is similarly elevated and incised. A small retractor, 3 mm in width, is inserted into the inguinal canal and the cremaster muscles are bluntly separated from the shelving edge of the inguinal ligament. After these maneuvers, the spermatic cord surrounded by the cremaster muscles can be identified just beneath the incision.

Minimally Invasive Repair of Inguinal Hernias in Children

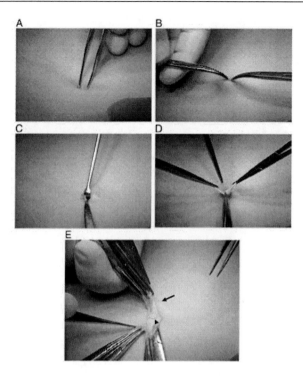

Figure 8. The selective sac extraction method (SSEM) in a male patient. The hernia sac is selectively extracted from an extremely small incision (A-D). The sac is opened and transected (D-E). The proximal part of the sac (black arrow) is freed as highly as possible before ligation, and the vas is shown at the bottom of the proximal sac (arrowhead) (E) (Reprinted from J Pediatr Surg, Ikeda H, et al. A selective sac extraction method: another minimally invasive procedure for inguinal hernia repair in children: a technical innovation with satisfactory surgical and cosmetic results. J Pediatr Surg 2009; 44:1666-1671, with permission from Elsevier).

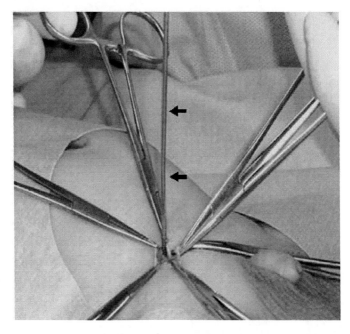

Figure 9. After the neck of the proximal sac is freed highly enough, a probe (arrows) inserted into the sac points in the direction of the pelvis and stands perpendicularly, indicating that the internal inguinal ring is just beneath the wound.

In the SSEM, the entire cord structure is not pulled out of the wound. After the cremaster muscles are partly elevated, the internal spermatic fascia is identified between cremasteric muscle fibers. The hernia sac is identified by dissecting the fascia anterocranially. The surrounding muscular and fascial tissues are teased and pulled bluntly down and away. By pushing back the muscular and fascial tissues into the wound, the hernia sac can be selectively extracted from the small wound. Then, the sac is opened and transected. The internal inguinal ring is confirmed by probing, and the distal part of the sac is pushed back into the inguinal canal by pulling the scrotum and testis. Now, only the proximal part of the sac is selectively extracted from the wound and can be freed as proximally as possible. The level where the sac is highly ligated is determined by identifying the preperitoneal fat tissue. After the neck of the sac is freed highly enough, a probe inserted into the proximal sac points in the direction of the pelvis (stands perpendicularly) and indicates that the internal inguinal ring is just beneath the wound (Figure 9). The vas and the testicular vessels are seen at the bottom of the proximal sac without exposing their entire length. A limited dissection of the vas and the vessels minimizes damage to these structures. If the vas and the testicular vessels are not identified, the skin incision is extended by a millimeter or so. At minimum , the vas should be identified before the neck of the sac is doubly ligated with unabsorbable sutures. After high ligation of the sac, the wound is closed.

SSEM Procedure in Female Patients

The procedure is fundamentally the same as that in male patients. A small incision is made where the hernia sac is felt passing over the pectineal line by palpation. The inguinal canal is opened and the internal oblique muscles are separated from the inguinal ligament. The hernia sac is identified between muscle fibers. The surrounding muscle fibers are bluntly pulled down and pushed back into the wound. The entire sac is selectively extracted from the wound and opened to confirm the round ligament. The presence or absence of ovary or fallopian tube sliding is confirmed. The proximal end of the sac is doubly ligated without transecting the hernia sac. The length of the wound can be further minimized if the sac is transected with the round ligament and the distal sac is pushed back into the inguinal canal before freeing the proximal sac, as highly as possible. However, this method is not usually adopted for fear that transection of the round ligament may cause complications such as uterine retroversion. After ligation of the proximal sac, the entire sac is pushed back into the inguinal canal and the procedure is completed by closing the wound.

Technical Feasibility of SSEM: A Retrospective Analysis

SSEM is an innovative technique in which only the hernia sac is selectively extracted from the wound instead of elevating the entire cord structures. In female patients, the round ligament is elevated and the hernia sac is extracted without pulling the surrounding muscular and fascial tissues out of the wound. The hernia, therefore, can be repaired through an extremely small skin incision. Injuries to the vas and testicular vessels are avoidable because their entire lengths are not exposed.

The technical feasibility of SEEM was retrospectively examined in 162 consecutive hernia repairs in which the SSEM was applied. Incarcerated or irreducible hernia, hernia with palpable ovary at repair, and hernia associated with an undescended testis were excluded from the indication of SSEM. The SSEM was successful in 92% of repairs. The incision lengths at the end of the procedure were less than 10 mm in these repairs. The success rate was 88% in repairs of male patients and 96% in females. In 8% of repairs, the procedure was converted to a conventional open method, Potts' operation, by extending the incision to 10 mm or longer. The reasons for conversion included a huge or thickened sac that could not be extracted from a small incision, obesity and thick subcutaneous tissue characteristics of early infancy, malpositioning of the skin incision, and difficulty in sac identification. The median length of incision at the end of repairs in male patients was 7.5 mm, whereas the length in female patients was 6.5 mm. With a median follow-up time of 20 months (range, 12 to 29 months), there was no recurrence of inguinal hernia. No parents reported postoperative complications such as wound infection, testicular atrophy, or testicular translocation. More than 90% of the parents rated wound cosmesis as good or excellent. Consequently, it was concluded that inguinal hernia repair with SSEM through a minimal skin incision was technically feasible with very satisfactory surgical and cosmetic results.

SSEM as a Standard approach

As described above, laparoscopic repairs have a marked advantage when contralateral exploration is indicated. However, there is an ongoing discussion regarding the necessity of routine contralateral exploration and surgery for a PPV. If surgery for a PPV is not supported and contralateral exploration is abandoned, the advantage of laparoscopic repairs compared to conventional open repairs is limited to a better wound cosmesis. On the other hand, the SSEM was devised as a modification of conventional open repair in order to achieve excellent wound cosmesis. Laparoscopy is unnecessary and laparoscopy-related complications can be avoided by using SSEM. Since a retrospective study has shown that the surgical and cosmetic results of SSEM are excellent, it has the potential to become the standard procedure for inguinal hernia repair in children. To confirm the safety and usefulness of the procedure, a prospective study is now being conducted.

References

[1] Russel RH. The etiology and treatment of inguinal hernia in the young. *Lancet*, 1899; 2:1353-1358.
[2] Banks WM. On the radical cure of hernia, by removal of the sac and stitching together the pillars of the ring. *Br. Med. J.* 1882; 985-988.
[3] Potts WJ, Riker WL, Lewis JE. The treatment of inguinal hernia in infants and children. *Ann. Surg.* 1950; 132:566-576.
[4] Sachs M, Damm M, Encke A. Historical evolution of inguinal hernia repair. *World. J. Surg.* 1997; 21:218-223.
[5] Turner P. The radical cure of inguinal hernia in children. *Proc. R. Soc. Med.* 1912; 5:133-140.
[6] Russell RH. Inguinal hernia and operative procedure. *Surg. Gynecol. Obstet*, 1925; 41:605-609.
[7] Herzfeld G. Hernia in infancy. *Am. J. Surg.* 1938; 39:422-428.
[8] Coles JS. Operative cure of inguinal hernia in infancy and childhood. *Am. J. Surg.* 1945; 69:366-371.
[9] Yatsushiro T. Treatment of inguinal hernia in children (in Japanese). Juntendo Iji Kenkyukai Zasshi 1911; 457:1-10.
[10] Kurlan MZ, Wels PB, Piedad OH. Inguinal herniorrhaphy by the Mitchell Banks Technique. *J. Pediatr. Surg.* 1972; 4:427-429.
[11] White JJ, Haller Jr. JA. Groin hernia in infants and children. In: Nyhus LM, Condon RE, editors. Hernia. Philadelphia, PA: Lippincott; 1978; 101-136.
[12] Griffith CA. The Marcy repair of indirect inguinal hernia. In: Nyhus LM, Condon RE, editors. Hernia. Philadelphia, PA: Lippincott; 1978; 137-162.
[13] Schier F, Montupet P, Esposito C. Laparoscopic inguinal herniorrhaphy in children: a three-center experience with 933 repairs. *J. Pediatr. Surg.* 2002; 37:395-397.
[14] Schier F. Laparoscopic inguinal hernia repair – a prospective personal series of 542 children. *J. Pediatr. Surg.* 2006; 41:1081-1084.
[15] Giseke S, Glass M, Tapadar P, et al. A true laparoscopic herniotomy in children: evaluation of long-term outcome. *J. Laparoendosc. Adv. Surg. Tech.* 2010; 20:191-194.
[16] Takehara H, Yakabe S, Kameoka K. Laparoscopic percutaneous extraperitoneal closure for inguinal hernia in children: clinical outcome of 972 repairs done in 3 pediatric surgical institutions. *J. Pediatr. Surg.* 2006; 41:1999-2003.

[17] Rothenberg RE, Barnett T. Bilateral herniotomy in infants and children. *Surgery*, 1955; 37:947-950.
[18] Sparkman RS. Bilateral exploration in inguinal hernia in juvenile patients. *Surgery*, 1962; 51:393-406.
[19] Muraji T, Noda T, Higashimoto Y, et al. Contralateral incidence after repair of unilateral inguinal hernia in infants and children. *Pediatr. Surg. Int.* 1993; 8:455-457.
[20] Surana R, Puri P. Is contralateral exploration necessary in infants with unilateral inguinal hernia? *J. Pediatr. Surg.* 1993; 28:1026-1027.
[21] Ulman I, Demircan M, Arikan A, et al. Unilateral inguinal hernia in girls: is routine contralateral exploration justified? *J. Pediatr. Surg.* 1995; 30:1684-1686.
[22] Kemmotsu H, Oshima Y, Joe K, et al. The features of contralateral manifestations after the repair of unilateral inguinal hernia. *J. Pediatr. Surg.* 1998; 33:1099-1103.
[23] Tackett LD, Breuer CK, Luks FI, et al. Incidence of contralateral inguinal hernia: a prospective analysis. *J. Pediatr. Surg.* 1999; 34:684-688.
[24] Ikeda H, Suzuki N, Takahashi A, et al. Risk of contralateral manifestation in children with unilateral inguinal hernia: should hernia in children be treated contralaterally? *J. Pediatr. Surg.* 2000; 35:1746-1748.
[25] Miltenburg DM, Nuchtern JG, Jaksic T, et al. Meta-analysis of the risk of metachronous hernia in infants and children. *Am. J. Surg.* 1997; 174:741-744.
[26] Ron O, Eaton S, Pierro A. Systematic review of the risk of developing a metachronous contralateral inguinal hernia in children. *Br. J. Surg.* 2007; 94:804-811.
[27] Manoharan S, Samarakkody U, Kulkarni M, et al. Evidence-based change of practice in the management of unilateral inguinal hernia. *J. Pediatr. Surg.* 2005; 40:1163-1166.
[28] Rowe MI, Copelson LW, Clatworthy HW. The patent processus vaginalis and the inguinal hernia. *J. Pediatr. Surg.* 1969; 4:102-107.
[29] Chin T, Liu C, Wei C. The morphology of the contralateral internal inguinal rings is age-dependent in children with unilateral inguinal hernia. *J. Pediatr. Surg.* 1995; 30:1663-1665.
[30] Powell RW. Intraoperative diagnostic pneumoperitoneum in pediatric patients with unilateral inguinal hernias: the Goldstein test. *J. Pediatr. Surg.* 1985; 20:418-421.

[31] Downey EC, Maher DP, Thompson WR. Diagnostic pneumoperitoneum accurately predicts the presence of patent processus vaginalis. *J. Pediatr. Surg.* 1995; 30:1271-1272.
[32] Wulkan ML, Wiener ES, VanBalen N, et al. Laparoscopy through the open ipsilateral sac to evaluate presence of contralateral hernia. *J. Pediatr. Surg.* 1996; 31:1174-1177.
[33] Miltenburg DM, Nuchtern JG, Jaksic T, et al. Laparoscopic evaluation of the pediatric inguinal hernia – a meta-analysis. *J. Pediatr. Surg.* 1998; 33:874-879.
[34] Mollen KP, Kane TD. Inguinal hernia: what we have learned from laparoscopic evaluation of the contralateral side. *Curr. Opin. Pediatr.* 2007; 19:344-348.
[35] Antonoff MB, Kreykes NS, Saltzman DA, et al. American Academy of Pediatric Section on Surgery hernia survey revisited. *J. Pediatr. Surg.* 2005; 40:1009-1014.
[36] Tamaddon H, Phillips JD, Nakayama DK. Laparoscopic evaluation of the contralateral groin in pediatric inguinal hernia patients: a comparison of 70- and 120-degree endoscopes. *J. Laparoendosc. Adv. Surg. Tech.* 2005; 15:653-660.
[37] Sözübir S, Ekingen G, Şenel U, et al. A continuous debate on contralateral processus vaginalis: evaluation technique and approach to patency. *Hernia,* 2006; 10:74-78.
[38] Maddox MM, Smith DP. A long-term prospective analysis of pediatric unilateral inguinal hernias: should laparascopy or anything else influence the management of the contralateral side? *J. Pediatr. Urol.* 2008; 4:141-145.
[39] Zamakhshardy M, Ein A, Ein SH, et al. Predictors of metachronous inguinal hernias in children. *Pediatr. Surg. Int.* 2009; 25:69-71.
[40] El-Gohary HA. Laparoscopic ligation of inguinal hernia in girls. *Pediatr. Endosurg. Innov. Tech.* 1997; 1:185-188.
[41] Bharathi RS, Arora M, Baskaran V. Minimal access surgery of pediatric inguinal hernias: a review. *Surg. Endosc.* 2008; 22:1751-1762.
[42] Schier F. Laparoscopic herniorrhaphy in girls. *J. Pediatr. Surg.* 1998; 33:1495-1497.
[43] Montupet P, Esposito C. Laparoscopic treatment of congenital inguinal hernia in children. *J. Pediatr. Surg.* 1999; 34:420-423.

[44] Shalaby RY, Fawy M, Soliman SM, et al. A new simplified technique for needlescopic inguinal herniorrhaphy in children. *J. Pediatr. Surg.* 2006; 41:863-867.
[45] Yip KF, Tam PKH, Li MKW. Laparoscopic flip-flap hernioplasty: an innovative technique for pediatric hernia surgery. *Surg. Endosc.* 2004; 18:1126-1129.
[46] Hassan ME, Mustafawi AR. Laparoscopic flip-flap technique versus conventional inguinal hernia repair in children. *JSLS,* 2007; 11:90-93.
[47] Riquelme M, Aranda A, Riquelme-Q M. Laparoscopic pediatric inguinal hernia repair: no ligation, just resection. *J. Laparoendosc. Adv. Surg. Tech.* 2010; 20:77-80.
[48] Endo M, Ukiyama E. Laparoscopic closure of patent processus vaginalis in girls with inguinal hernia using a specially devised suture needle. *Pediatr. Endosurg. Innov. Tech.* 2001; 5:187-191.
[49] Endo M, Watanabe T, Nakano M, et al. Laparoscopic completely extraperitoneal repair of inguinal hernia in children: a single-institute experience with 1,257 repairs compared with cut-down herniorrhaphy. *Surg. Endosc.* 2009; 23:1706-1712.
[50] Lee Y, Liang J. Experience with 450 cases of micro-laparoscopic herniotomy in infants and children. *Pediatr. Endosurg. Innov. Tech.* 2002; 6:25-28.
[51] Harrison MR, Lee H, Albanese CT, et al. Subcutaneous endoscopically assisted ligation (SEAL) of the internal ring for repair of inguinal hernias in children: a novel technique. *J. Pediatr. Surg.* 2005; 40:1177-1180.
[52] Ozgediz D, Roayaie K, Lee H, et al. Subcutaneous endoscopically assisted ligation (SEAL) of the internal ring for repair of inguinal hernias in children: report of a new technique and early results. *Surg. Endosc.* 2007; 21:1327-1331.
[53] Tam YH, Lee KH, Sihoe JDY, et al. Laparoscopic hernia repair in children by the hook method: a single-center series of 433 consecutive patients. *J. Pediatr. Surg.* 2009; 44:1502-1505.
[54] Chan KL, Hui WC, Tam PKH. Prospective, randomized, single-center, single-blinded comparison of laparoscopic vs open repair of pediatric inguinal hernia. *Surg. Endosc.* 2005; 19:927-932.
[55] Rescorla FJ: Hernias and Umbilicus, in Oldham KT, Colombani PM, Foglia RP, Skinner MA (eds): Principles and Practice of Pediatric Surgery, Philadelphia, PA, Lippincott Williams and Wilkins, 2005, pp 1087-1101.

[56] Chan KL, Chan HY, Tam PKH. Towards a near-zero recurrence rate in laparoscopic inguinal hernia repair for pediatric patients of all ages. *J. Pediatr. Surg.* 2007; 42:1993-1997.
[57] Treef W, Schier F. Characteristics of laparoscopic inguinal hernia recurrences. *Pediatr. Surg. Int.* 2009; 25:149-152.
[58] Marte A, Sabatino MD, Borrelli M, et al. Decreased recurrence rate in the laparoscopic herniorrhaphy in children: comparison between two techniques. *J. Laparoendosc. Adv. Surg. Tech.* 2009; 19:259-262.
[59] Bharathi RS, Arora M, Baskaran V. Pediatric inguinal hernia: laparoscopic versus open surgery. *JSLS,* 2008; 12:277-281.
[60] Koivusalo AI, Korpela R, Wirtavuori K, et al. A single-blinded, randomized comparison of laparoscopic versus open hernia repair in children. *Pediatrics,* 2009; 123:332-337.
[61] Tsai YC, Wu C, Yang SS. Open versus minilaparoscopic herniorrhaphy for children: a prospective comparative trial with midterm follow-up evaluation. *Surg. Endosc.* 2010; 24:21-24.
[62] IPEG guidelines for inguinal hernia and hydrocele. *J. Laparoendosc. Adv. Surg .Tech.* 2010; 20:x-xiv.
[63] Clarke S. Pediatric inguinal hernia and hydrocele: an evidence-based review in the era of minimal access surgery. *J. Laparoendosc. Adv. Surg. Tech.* 2010; 20:305-309.
[64] Ikeda H, Hatanaka M, Suzuki M, et al. A selective sac extraction method: another minimally invasive procedure for inguinal hernia repair in children: a technical innovation with satisfactory surgical and cosmetic results. *J. Pediatr. Surg.* 2009; 44:1666-1671.

In: Hernias: Types, Symptoms and Treatment
Editor: James H. Wagner

ISBN: 978-1-61324-125-7
© 2011 Nova Science Publishers, Inc.

Chapter 2

Surgical Approach to Parastomal Hernias

V.B. Tsirline, I. Belyansky, D.A. Klima, K.L. Harold and B.T. Heniford[*]

Division of Gastrointestinal and Minimally Invasive Surgery, Carolinas Laparoscopic and Advanced Surgery Program, Carolinas Medical Center Charlotte, North Carolina, USA

Abstract

Parastomal hernia is an incisional abdominal wall hernia that involves a stoma. It is a common problem in patients with an intestinal stoma with an incidence of up to 50% or more.

Patients with stomas are at the highest risk of herniation during the initial 3-5 years after surgery, although hernia occurrence has been reported as late as 20 years after stoma creation. Herniation usually develops lateral to the stoma site.

Once a parastomal hernia has been diagnosed, seventy percent of the patients will be asymptomatic and can be managed nonoperatively. Typical

---

[*] 1025 Morehead Medical Drive, Suit 300, Charlotte, NC 28204, Phone (704)355-3168, Fax (704) 355-4117, E-mail: todd.heniford@carolinas.org

reasons for surgical intervention include bowel obstruction, bowel strangulation, bleeding, pain, and poor fit of the stoma appliance.

Surgical therapy includes direct tissue repair of the defect, stoma relocation, and placement of a prosthetic mesh. Irrespective of technique, open repair is associated with high morbidity and non-mesh repair carries a high recurrence rate.

For local tissue repair of parastomal hernias and stoma relocation, recurrence is seen in 46 to 100% and 76% respectively. When utilizing prosthetics, a keyhole mesh configuration and nonslit mesh repairs have been described. Dr Sugarbaker first described the nonslit mesh repair in 1980; this technique has been most effective, with the lowest recurrence rate.

The success of the Sugarbaker repair is attributed to the flap-valve action of the mesh on the bowel as it exits the peritoneal cavity and enters the abdominal wall. Minimally invasive approaches to parastomal hernia repair have gained popularity.

Mancini et al. described their experience with a laparoscopic modified Sugarbaker technique; patients were followed for 19 months and had a recurrence rate of 4%.

A review of literature supports the use of minimally invasive approach with prosthetic reinforcement as the optimal means of parastomal hernia repair.

History

In modern surgery, ostomy creation is a common procedure used to divert the enteral contents for variety of clinical conditions. In 1776, Pillore performed the first documented cecostomy on a wine merchant with an obstructing rectal cancer [1]. The procedure was initially a success, as the patient's bowels were decompressed, but death followed 28 days later due to swallowed quicksilver. Although, the concept and the case report of the procedure were described earlier, it is thought that colostomy had its real birth in 1793, when Duret performed a successful descending colostomy on a 3-day old infant with imperforate anus [1, 2].

Today ostomy creation is a widely performed procedure and includes enterostomies, ileal conduits, cecostomies, and various types of colostomies. Parastomal hernia is the most common late complication of a surgical stoma [2-4]. Parastomal hernias have been described as early as stomas, so much so that many experts consider parastomal herniation an inevitable consequence of colostomy creation [5], while others regard it as an incisional hernia at the site of the stoma [6].

Risk Factors

Chronically elevated intra-abdominal pressure and poor connective tissue integrity are some of the most important physiological factors responsible for the late development of abdominal wall hernias [7-11]. Risk factors for parastomal hernias include older age, obesity, diabetes, pulmonary disease involving chronic cough, malnutrition, steroid use, as well as a history of previous abdominal hernia and wound sepsis [10, 11]. Additionally, inflammatory bowel disease appears to be associated with an increased incidence of stoma complications including eventration and parastomal hernia [12-14]. While all of these factors are thought to predispose patients to stoma complications, in multi-factorial analysis only age and abdominal diameter (as a surrogate marker of increased intraabdominal pressure) were independently linked to the risk of parastomal hernia [15-17].

Parastomal hernia repair presents a surgical challenge, as the presence of a functional bowel passing through the defect makes it impossible to restore the fascial continuity. Surgical therapy includes direct tissue repair of the defect, stoma relocation, and placement of a prosthetic mesh. However, there is not a single method that all experts in the field unanimously agree upon, as there is lack of prospective randomized studies to compare their efficacy. Most of the currently performed repairs are still associated with high hernia recurrence rates as well as other complications. With the number of bowel diversions on the rise [18], general surgeons need to address parastomal defects more often than before. This chapter reviews issues associated with parastomal hernias and different methods that have been employed for their repair.

Incidence

The incidence of parastomal hernias varies by ostomy type, anatomic location, construction technique, and patient characteristics. In early reports a paracolostomy hernia was noted from 2 to 20 percent of the time [6, 19-21], while life-table analysis suggests a rate of 37 percent [10]. Ileal conduits for urinary diversion and ileostomies appear to have a similar frequency of parastomal herniation as other ostomies [22-26], although this is an area of debate, with some authors suggesting that paracolostomy hernias are more common due to the larger fascial defect required to admit the colon [10]. Likewise, there is mixed evidence on whether loop ileostomies have lower herniation rates than loop colostomies [21, 27, 28]. Patients are at the highest risk of herniation during the initial 3-5 years after the surgery [10, 15], although hernia occurrence has been reported as far out as 20-30 years after stoma creation [29]. Like ventral and incisional hernias the rate of parastomal hernias increases with time [15, 30].

The widespread use of Computed Tomography (CT) scanning has lead to the increased detection of small asymptomatic parastomal hernias [31], with recent studies suggesting that the actual incidence of parastomal hernias may be 52% or higher [22, 32, 33]. With lack of a uniform definition of a parastomal hernia, variation in technique, and wide range of follow-ups, the true rate of parastomal hernias is difficult to estimate, but most experts believe that it falls between 30% and 50% in a general surgical practice [2].

Classification and Diagnosis

Depending on the abdominal wall region where the ostomy was placed, different types of parastomal hernias may develop. Devlin and Kingsnorth classified parastomal defects into four subtypes [34]:

1. subcutaneous type – subcutaneous hernia sac
2. interstitial type – hernia sac within the muscle/aponeurotic layers of the abdomen
3. peristomal type – bowel prolapsing through a circumferential hernia sac enclosing the stoma
4. intrastomal type – hernia sac between the intestinal wall and the everted intestinal layer

Herniation usually develops lateral to the stoma site [35, 36], most commonly in the subcutaneous space (Type 1) [34]. Classifying parastomal hernias on a physical exam may be challenging, as they can range from nearly undetectable to quite large. Advanced imaging studies such as abdominal Computed Tomography with enteral contrast may be advantageous in differentiating between the types of defects [37]. Unfortunately, the formal criteria for clinical diagnosis are lacking [2] and few published studies explicitly describe the criteria used in their patient follow-up. Some authors classify all palpable defects adjacent to the stoma site as herniation [33, 38]; however, parastomal bulges may represent a spectrum of pathology from stretching of the abdominal wall fascia to stomal prolapse. Appropriately diagnosing a parastomal hernia type does not necessarily alter the patient management, as there is no literature to suggest that any of the above subtypes differ clinically in terms of patient symptoms, risk of complications, or repair technique. Although the type of parastomal hernia may not be clinically relevant, it is essential to differentiate a parastomal hernia from a stomal prolapse before proceeding with surgery, since the methods of repair are quite different. In a Cochrane Review, parastomal hernias were defined as a formation of a hernia beside the stoma, and ostomy prolapse was defined as an eversion of the stoma through the abdominal wall [27].

Several studies make a distinction between parastomal hernia and prolapse during follow-up [39, 40], however, formal clinical assessment guidelines are lacking. Taking a detailed history and performing a thorough physical exam is paramount. In their work, Williams and colleagues illustrated that a parastomal herniation can be clinically diagnosed by making the patient cough or valsalva, while performing a digital examination of the ostomy [31]. In the presence of a parastomal hernia, this maneuver may aid in identifying a bulge by digital exam, and is termed a "cough impulse" at the stoma site [31]. When in doubt, abdominal CT may aid in confirming the diagnosis [37].

Stoma prolapse can be distressing to the patient, but is usually of no functional significance. While prolapse has been reported in up to 25% of cases, incarceration and strangulation are rare [4]. Topical osmotic therapy with sugar to shrink an edematous incarcerated prolapse often allows bowel reduction; otherwise the prolapse may be treated with a local resection of the distal redundant bowel and reconstruction at the mucocutaneous junction [4].

Prevention of Parastomal Hernias

Since stoma construction is associated with a high frequency of parastomal defects, great efforts have been put forth to identify the optimal surgical method of the initial stoma construction that would prevent future herniation. Unfortunately, the solution to this surgical dilemma remains to be found, as prospective randomized studies have not been performed. Although most of the current practices are based on retrospective and some prospective data, it is clear that several surgical concepts and guidelines must be kept in mind when fashioning a stoma.

The field of stoma surgery has significantly evolved since the first report of a successful colostomy construction. As the concept gained popularity, a variety of methods were described, including stomas placement through the laparotomy incision, the umbilical region, the lateral abdominal muscle compartments, the rectus muscle, and even through the lumbar region [1].

Clearly, most of the earlier choices were based on surgeon preference and ingenuity, as these decisions were usually guided by practical intra-operative considerations such as the mobility of the distal segment of the bowel available to construct a "neo-anus" and its intra-abdominal position in relation to the abdominal wall [1].

Interestingly, umbilical stoma construction was associated with lower morbidity rates than lateral stomas, and this method was utilized more frequently in the days when surgeons routinely used paramedian abdominal incisions [1]. This practice changed when midline laparotomy incisions were found to be superior, especially for emergent operations requiring four-quadrant exploration, and became commonplace [1].

Construction of a stoma through the laparotomy incision is strongly discouraged in adults, as this has been shown to result in catastrophic rates of wound infection, dehiscence, and herniation [41, 42]. Several retrospective studies found lower rates of parastomal herniation with extraperitoneal colostomies [10, 43, 44], however, others have challenged these findings [45] and this method has not received widespread acceptance among surgeons. With the advent of minimally invasive techniques, some surgeons strongly advocate laparoscopic ostomy construction [46], however, the role of laparoscopy in lowering the incidence of parastomal hernias has not been reported with sufficient follow-up [47].

On the other hand, it was noted (though never proven in a randomized study) that placement of the stoma through the rectus abdominis muscle and making a smaller fascial aperture may be important intra-operative technical decisions that decrease the frequency of parastomal hernias. For this reason, we discuss these techniques in greater detail below.

Stoma Placement through Rectus Abdominis Muscle

Many surgeons believe that bringing out a stoma through the rectus abdominis muscle as opposed to the lateral abdominal compartments will minimizes the subsequent chance of a parastomal hernia. This concept can be understood by looking at the anatomy of the lateral abdominal muscles (external oblique, internal oblique and transversus abdominis), where several avascular planes exist between the aponeurotic layers of the abdominal muscle. As the bowel traverses the lateral muscle components these planes form potential spaces that may house a hernia sac. In contrast, placing the stoma directly through the rectus abdominis muscle may decrease the risk of herniation because no such planes exist within the rectus sheath. When performing trans-rectus abdominis ostomy pull-through the rectus muscle should not be divided, but rather split vertically so as to provide muscular reinforcement of the stoma. This technique of preserving the rectus muscle allows it to contract during abdominal flexion preventing intra-abdominal viscera from herniating through it along the distal limb of the stoma.

While there are no randomized trials to address the utility of this technique, several retrospective reviews totaling over 200 patients have shown parastomal herniation rates of 1-3% for stomas brought out through the rectus muscle, nearly ten-fold lower than 19-22% herniation of stomas placed lateral to the rectus muscle [2, 48]. These results are not uniformly supported by the available literature; as multiple retrospective studies failed to show a difference in outcomes between stoma locations [3, 10, 31, 49].

Despite the ongoing debate, many authors deem it prudent to construct stomas through the rectus abdominis muscle as there are no proven disadvantages of this approach and in most patients this corresponds to a favorable stoma position on the abdominal surface [4].

Aperture Size

Multiple studies have documented that larger fascial openings may be associated with an increased risk of parastomal herniation [45, 50]. Many authors suggest that the opening should be large enough to allow the bowel to pass through it but the diameter of the opening should be 2.5-3.0 cm for a colostomy and 1.5-2.0 cm for a small bowel conduit. Several reports attempted to justify these dimensions based on the physics of the abdominal wall tension applying La Place law, however, such considerations remain theoretical [45, 51]. The recommendations for stoma aperture have ranged from finger-based estimates [52, 53], to intestinal width based [54]. Introduction of mechanical cutting devices for aperture creation has yielded some favorable results [55], although no randomized studies are available. In a CT-based study of 28 patients with an end ileostomy, an aperture of 3 cm was associated with significantly more parastomal hernias (8 out of 9 patients) compared to an aperture of 2 cm (1 out of 17 patients) [3]. In the absence of further evidence on the optimal stoma size, authors advise the creation of the smallest opening that permits a viable stoma without ischemia [3]. There is no evidence that sewing the bowel mesentery to the fascia reduces parastomal herniation [2], and doing so may actually result in inadvertent suture ligation of the blood supply to the ostomy resulting in ischemia.

Repair of Parastomal Hernias

Traditionally results in surgical repair of parastomal hernias were poor. Because many parastomal hernias are small and asymptomatic, much consideration was given to non-operative management of parastomal hernias and eventrations [4]. The absolute indications remain incarceration, obstruction, strangulation and bowel ischemia as well as perforation.

Today routine indications have expanded to include intermittent obstructive symptoms, local pain or irritation, aesthetic considerations, poor appliance fit and factors that may otherwise negatively impact the quality of life [11].

Approximately half a century of evolution of parastomal hernia repair techniques has seen several stages and considerable controversy among surgeons. While prosthetic reinforcement has proven superior to other techniques, the quest for the ultimate methodology for parastomal hernia repair continues as long-term recurrence rates remain in the double digits in the best of hands.

Primary Repair

In 1965 Thorlakson described the technique of primary fascial repair of parastomal hernias [35]. A peristomal incision is made approximately 5 cm away from the mucocutaneous junction over the region of the hernia defect. The dissection is carried down adjacent to the stoma onto the hernia sac. The sac is mobilized and the hernia is reduced into the abdomen. The fascial edges are sewn together loosely with non-absorbable suture.

This local repair approach is attractive because it is fast, easy to perform, and avoids a formal laparotomy. Unfortunately, this method places the reconstructed fascial layers under tension. When addressing a parastomal hernia for the first time, this approach has a failure rate of 46%, and when dealing with a recurrent defect the failure rate is as high as 100% [56]. In 1997 Bewes described a case report of a modified local tissue repair of a parastomal hernia. This method utilized a fascial "rotation flap" in order to reduce the tension in the fascia [57].

Although primary repair of parastomal fascial defects may have a role in select situations when prosthetic materials are contraindicated or unavailable, it is otherwise not recommended due to unacceptably high failure rates [29, 58, 59].

Stoma Relocation

Stoma relocation may be performed with or without a formal laparotomy. This approach is especially useful if the stoma position is suboptimal from the medical or maintenance standpoint [3, 60].

Studies involving stoma relocation for parastomal hernia repair have reported a wide range of outcomes. The advantages of stoma relocation without a laparotomy include shorter operating times, less postoperative pain, avoiding extensive adhesiolysis and subsequent adhesion formation [61-63]. The overall integrity of the abdominal wall is better preserved and there are significantly fewer post-operative midline incisional hernias, intra-abdominal adhesions and related complications [58, 64].

Stoma relocation implies creating the second fascial defect and closure of the original defect. These mechanical defects may be quite large, as they are compounded by years of non-uniform fascial stretching and their primary closures are technically difficult to perform in a tension-free fashion, with some requiring the use of prosthetic material to reconstruct the fascial continuity.

Some authors advocate a technique of incising the cutaneous portion of the previous midline laparotomy scar and raising a flap toward the hernia sac in order to assess the size of the defect. This approach is flexible in providing adequate exposure for local repair with an option of converting to a formal laparotomy at the surgeon's discretion [65, 66].

Stoma relocation carries at least as high of a hernia recurrence rate as the original operation, and the risk grows with each subsequent operation [56]. By the most optimistic estimates the hernia recurrence rates with stoma relocation are lower than those for primary defect repair, and probably range from 30 to 50%, however, these repair failure rates remain unacceptable as a long-term solution.

Mesh Repair: Pros and Cons

In 1955, the introduction of polypropylene mesh dramatically reduced recurrence rates for incisional hernia repairs [67]. It is widely accepted that a tension free approach is the key to a durable and robust repair. Although the use of mesh has drastically improved the outcomes of abdominal wall hernia surgery, experience showed that it is associated with a unique set of complications. Indeed, the use of prosthetic implants can be a double-edged sword, with the risk of seeding the mesh with microorganisms intraoperatively [68], resulting in a mesh infection that may require another operation to remove the source [69-72]. Aside from the technical failure to create a tension free repair, wound infection is the most important factor contributing to the hernia recurrence [9]. When mesh is used in a clean incisional hernia case along with a prophylactic dose of an antibiotic, the infection rate is 1-2% [73, 74]; this rate may be higher in a parastomal hernia repair case. With the liberal use of prosthetics for abdominal wall hernias, the adverse effects of mesh contact with the intra-abdominal organs became evident. A concern for bowel erosion caused some reluctance to use synthetic materials around the stoma [67], but high failure rates of primary repair demanded a change in practice. The concern of bowel erosion was addressed by multiple authors, and several published methods have emphasized the importance of leaving a 2-3 mm gap around the bowel limb to prevent mesh contact with the serosa [65, 75, 76]. Some authors described special techniques of fascial mobilization to protect the bowel from the encircling mesh [77]. Interestingly, to date, very few cases of erosion of the stoma limb by the surrounding polypropylene mesh have been reported [78]. In a series of 58 patients undergoing parastomal hernia repair with mesh, Steel et al. reported only 1 mesh erosion, which was managed *without* mesh excision [79]. Although special technical emphasis should be placed on ensuring that mesh is not too tight around the stoma, based on the available literature one can conclude that mesh repair of parastomal hernias is fairly safe and its use is necessary to reduce recurrences.

Choice of Prosthetic Materials

A variety of synthetic and biologic materials have been employed [80-89] in the repair of abdominal wall hernias. Prior to the advent of polypropylene, titanium wires were used for hernia repairs, which led to significant restriction of abdominal wall mobility. In the late 1950s polypropylene mesh became the gold standard prosthetic material for hernia repair reinforcement [67] and subsequently for parastomal hernia repair [90].

With the shift to the intraperitoneal onlay repair with wide fascial overlap, the two major disadvantages of polypropylene became clinically apparent: mesh shrinkage leading to recurrences and intestinal adhesions causing bowel obstructions and mesh erosion into bowel threatening an intra-abdominal catastrophe [91-93].

In addressing these issues polytetrafluoroethylene (ePTFE) was favored. Mechanically ePTFE is similar to synthetic clothing and has lower bioavailability causing almost no bowel adhesions and reduced contraction over time [80, 81]. This material has poor memory and lacks rigidity which can be argued as optimal or suboptimal for abdominal fascial reinforcement, especially in when used in the keyhole repair of parastomal hernias [94].

Newer synthetic polymers including polyester (Parietex) [86], polyvinylidene fluoride (Dynamesh) [82, 95], lightweight polypropylene [96, 97], as well as composite meshes (combination products) have been used [98]. Each of these materials has its own set of advantages and drawbacks. Collagen matrix based biologic meshes have been promoted for their possible efficacy in infected fields, and potential better host tissue integration than their synthetic counterparts [85, 88, 89, 99], although this has not been proven.

Overall, biologic meshes may allow the host to eradicate low bacterial loads of up to 10^4 colony forming units (CFU) but become rapidly integrated into the tissues while losing their tensile strength [REFERNECE YOURSELVES]. However, moderate infection challenges (10^6 CFU) of the biologic mesh lead to infection, as reflected by the final bacterial counts, as do synthetic implants [100]. These grafts come with a high price tag and a theoretical risk of viral disease transmission. Additionally, these grafts often do not maintain their mechanical strength long-term, resulting in higher repair failure rates than synthetics.

Most recently the use of lightweight polypropylene combined with absorbable synthetics has been shown to be able to provide durable long-term reinforcement, moderate tissue integration, lesser degree of mesh contraction and bowel adhesions, and some resistance to infection [96, 97]. There is emerging evidence that antimicrobial-bound mesh may permit its use in infected surgical fields [REFENCE YOURSLEVES]. However, no randomized controlled trials are available to establish the superiority of a particular mesh type for repair of parastomal hernias [11].

Parastomal Hernia Mesh Repair

Since 1977, various prosthetic reinforced parastomal hernia repair methods have been described. These techniques focus on the differences in mesh implantation with respect to the abdominal fascia and include: onlay, sublay, and intraperitoneal placement [51, 65, 101-103]. An onlay mesh is placed superficial to the anterior fascia. A sublay mesh is placed between the rectus muscle and the posterior rectus fascia. With the intraperitoneal technique the mesh is introduced into the peritoneal cavity and secured to the abdominal wall in a keyhole or Sugarbaker fashion; the intraperitoneal methods are unique in that they can be performed using a laparoscopic approach.

A mention of the inlay technique is of historical interest, as this method has been described in repair of incisional hernias. This approach is associated with a high recurrence rate [2] and thus, it is a suboptimal repair choice for parastomal hernias. In this technique, the mesh is cut to the size of the defect and sutured to the fascial edges producing no fascial overlap; as a result this method has high failure rates. When using prosthetic reinforcement, an overlap of 5-10 cm in all directions is optimal, as postoperative mesh integration with the native fascia improves the durability of the repair [104].

Onlay Mesh

The general objective of the onlay repair is superficial reinforcement of the anterior abdominal fascia around the stoma. This approach is advantageous as it can be performed locally and often through a small incision, avoiding a laparotomy and minimizing the risk of incisional hernias. Early reports described making a circumferential incision, stapling off the stoma, then passing it through the center hole of a polypropylene mesh to be attached to the anterior fascia, followed by stoma reconstruction [90, 102, 105].

Leslie described an L-shaped incision around the stoma, starting along the previous laparotomy scar, in order to permit simultaneous incisional hernia repair, followed by polypropylene reinforcement of the fascia [11, 65, 106]. Tekkis described the technique of exposure through a lateral semicircular incision followed by 270° reinforcement of the parastomal fascia with polypropylene mesh [76]. Stoma relocation in combination with a prosthetic to cover both the old stoma site and reinforce the new stoma opening has also been described [107].

Sublay Mesh

Sublay mesh techniques for parastomal hernia are numerous. The mesh can be placed between the posterior rectus fascia and the rectus muscle [101], deep to the posterior fascia in the preperitoneal space [101], or intraperitoneally [108]. In the rest of this chapter we discuss several intraperitoneal mesh placement methods, as those are the more commonly used sublay techniques.

Intraperitoneal Onlay Mesh (IPOM)

In 1980, Sugarbaker was the first to describe the intraperitoneal onlay mesh (IPOM) technique [108]. Since then, this method has been modified and optimized to maximize its benefits as reported in several studies [80, 81, 109, 110], One of the advantages of the intraperitoneal approach is a wide exposure of the fascial defect from within the intraabdominal cavity, enabling the surgeon to place a large mesh with wide mesh-fascial overlap. The extent of overlap is important in providing a dynamic balance of forces on the mesh and an increase in surface area of mesh-to-fascia integration; these factors play an important role in the long-term durability of the repair. The intraperitoneally placed mesh prevents the intra-abdominal organs from entering the parastomal space and causing a hernia.

The disadvantages of the intraperitoneal approach include the need for a laparotomy, mesh contact with intestines, and the potential for contamination [75]. The initial skepticism has become less common with the advent of laparoscopic techniques and enhanced biomaterials to combat adhesions and infectious complications. The incidence of recurrence in open IPOM from pooled data has been estimated at 11% [2], however, there are significant differences in technique and complications between the individual reports. The two most widely used methods for mesh placement are the "Keyhole" and Sugarbaker technique.

Keyhole Technique

In order to place the mesh around the stoma without taking the stoma down, a slit is made between the edge of the mesh extending to the center trephine - this is known as the keyhole technique [111, 112]. The slit is usually sutured together. In 1992 Byers described the technique of intraperitoneal reinforcement with two parallel strips of polypropylene mesh sutured together around the colon [83]; this configuration of mesh was later modified to a keyhole. Despite refinements in technique [113] and better understanding of the biomaterials, the most recent studies quote a disappointing recurrence rate of 37 to 56% after the keyhole repair of parastomal hernias [94, 114].

The exact mechanism of recurrences is not entirely understood, but patient selection plays an important role, as patients with stomas are often cancer survivors with multiple comorbidities and poor tissue integrity resulting from chemotherapy. It is hypothesized that the fascial opening of the stoma widens over time allowing the passage of intra-abdominal structures along the externalized bowel. This is consistent with the observation that the recurrence after keyhole repair may be more common with highly pliable ePTFE mesh compared to the sturdy polypropylene-derived materials [94]. Mesh shrinkage may play a role as well by enlarging the central opening in the mesh [115].

Sugarbaker Technique

In 1985 Sugarbaker reported a series of 6 patients (with a total of 8 prior recurrences) undergoing parastomal hernia repair with a prosthetic mesh, where the bowel was tunneled superficial and lateral to the mesh rather than going through it [116]. The genius of this technique is that the "colon is led out through the mesh flap valve so that further herniation out around the colon is unlikely".

In the 4-7 years of follow-up there were no recurrences. Since then multiple series have reported successful utilization as well as modification of this technique with hernia rates of 0 to 33%. While the initial account described suturing the mesh to the fascial edges as an inlay, based on the evidence from ventral and incisional hernia repairs a 5cm fascial overlap [109] and transfascial fixation sutures [117] area employed resulting in a 4% overlap in a 25 patient series over a 4-38 month follow-up.

Laparoscopic IPOM

The first report of laparoscopic parastomal hernia repair used ePTFE mesh as a preperitoneal onlay patch with no slit [118]. Laparoscopic repair quickly gained popularity with various techniques and modifications [98, 111-113, 119-123]. In the four nonrandomized studies on laparoscopic IPOM technique the recurrence rate was 10% [2]. Because the laparoscopic approach avoids the laparotomy incision, there is no concern for subsequent incisional hernia - one of the major drawbacks of the open IPOM technique. However, laparoscopy is not always feasible in a reoperative abdomen, and conversion rates of 15% have been reported [124]. Intraoperative bowel injury - the dreaded complication of all hernia repairs involving mesh - was initially reported at higher rates of 22% in laparoscopic compared to open IPOM technique [98, 124]. More recent reports have shown decreased rates of complications as well as the possibility of conservative treatment in the face of mesh contamination. (You should add a couple better studies here, i.e. Craft, Harold, that have better outcomes)

Mesh Use at Stoma Creation

Parastomal hernias may occur in as many as 50% of the patients receiving colostomies, and some authors believe that they are almost inevitable given sufficient follow-up. Mesh-reinforced repair, while overwhelmingly successful in almost all other hernia types [7], has a much smaller impact on the parastomal hernia repairs, reducing the recurrence rates to 20-30% [94, 115, 125]. Therefore, prosthetic reinforcement has been suggested at the time of stoma creation [90]. One author reported no parastomal hernias after 4 years of follow-up in a study of 43 patients [103] with mesh placed during stoma formation, although one patient developed a stricture and required mesh removal. Parastomal hernia rates of under 8% were noted in other prospective series [126-128]. Intraperitoneal placement of mesh at the time of stoma creation has also been reported [129] with low morbidity and good results. Several randomized trials have shown promise in the use of synthetic and biologic mesh to reinforce the fascia during stoma creation [33, 130, 131], but small sample size limited their statistical power. Recently, a prospective randomized trial of 54 patients comparing conventional colostomy formation with stoma formation reinforced with UltraPro mesh showed 4.7% vs 50% hernia incidence at 1 year [38] and 13% vs 81% at 5 years [132] in favor of mesh reinforcement. Finally, a meta-analysis by Wijeyekoon et al. of three randomized trials found 12.3% vs 54.7% parastomal hernia rate (RR 0.23, 95% CI 0.06 to 0.81, $p < 0.02$) favoring prosthetic reinforcement of stomas at the initial operation. Apart from occasional stoma stenosis and one parastomal mesh?? infection, no additional or unusual complications have been reported with the use of mesh [133]. Formal comparisons showed no statistical differences in morbidity between conventional and mesh reinforced stomas [131]. There is compelling evidence that stoma construction with prosthetic reinforcement results in lower parastomal hernia rates and some authors propose that this should become the standard of care and further randomized trials should be discontinued [132]. To date there is no evidence of superiority of a particular material, synthetic or biologic, for fascial reinforcement during stoma creation or parastomal hernia repair.

Summary

Parastomal hernias have been around for as long as stomas themselves. They occur in at least half of patients, despite the surgeons' best efforts in making small fascial defects and bringing the stoma through the rectus abdominis muscle. At least one third of the parastomal hernias require surgical intervention due to symptoms ranging from discomfort to life-threatening complications. Detection of small asymptomatic hernias may be difficult, particularly their distinction from stoma prolapse, and imaging may aid in the diagnosis. Parastomal hernia repairs are flawed with high recurrence rates. Repair techniques have ranged from local primary repair (46-100% recurrence), to stoma relocation (30-60% recurrence), to prosthetic fascial reinforcement (20-50% recurrence) with or without a laparotomy. Intraperitoneal mesh placement is often performed laparoscopically using a keyhole or Sugarbaker techniques (37-56% and 0-33% recurrence rates respectively). A modified laparoscopic Sugarbaker technique with use of a composite or biologic mesh appears most promising, with the lowest rates of recurrence and minimal intraabdominal and wound complications. Mesh reinforcement during the initial stoma creation has been shown in randomized trials to result in significantly lower incidence of parastomal hernia (8-13%), while carrying the same morbidity as conventional stoma creation, and should be strongly considered. To date there is no evidence that one mesh or material type is superior to others for parastomal hernia repair.

References

[1] Dinnick, T., The origins and evolution of colostomy. *British Journal of Surgery*, 1934. 22(85): p. 142-154.
[2] Israelsson, L.A., Parastomal hernias. *Surg. Clin. North Am.* 2008. 88(1): p. 113-25, ix.
[3] Carne, P.W., G.M. Robertson, and F.A. Frizelle, Parastomal hernia. *Br. J. Surg.* 2003. 90(7): p. 784-93.
[4] Shellito, P.C., Complications of abdominal stoma surgery. *Dis. Colon. Rectum*. 1998. 41(12): p. 1562-72.
[5] Todd, I.P., *Intestinal Stomas*. 1978, London: William Heinemann Medical Books Ltd. 215.
[6] Pearl, R.K., Parastomal hernias. *World J. Surg.* 1989. 13(5): p. 569-72.
[7] Muschaweck, U., *Umbilical and epigastric hernia repair. Surg. Clin. North Am.* 2003. 83(5): p. 1207-21.
[8] Mislowsky, A., A. Hemphill, and D.V. Nasrallah, A scarless technique of umbilical hernia repair in the adult population. *Hernia*, 2008. 12(6): p. 627-30.
[9] Luijendijk, R.W., et al., Incisional hernia recurrence following "vest-over-pants" or vertical Mayo repair of primary hernias of the midline. *World J. Surg.* 1997. 21(1): p. 62-5; discussion 66.
[10] Londono-Schimmer, E.E., A.P. Leong, and R.K. Phillips, Life table analysis of stomal complications following colostomy. *Dis. Colon. Rectum.* 1994. 37(9): p. 916-20.
[11] Tadeo-Ruiz, G., et al., [Parastomal hernias: background, current status and future prospects]. *Cir. Esp.* 2010. 87(6): p. 339-49.
[12] Carlstedt, A., et al., Long-term ileostomy complications in patients with ulcerative colitis and Crohn's disease. *Int. J. Colorectal Dis.* 1987. 2(1): p. 22-5.

[13] Carlsen, E. and A. Bergan, Technical aspects and complications of end-ileostomies. *World J. Surg.* 1995. 19(4): p. 632-6.
[14] Saghir, J.H., et al., Factors that predict complications after construction of a stoma: a retrospective study. *Eur. J. Surg.* 2001. 167(7): p. 531-4.
[15] Mylonakis, E., et al., Life table analysis of hernia following end colostomy construction. *Colorectal Dis.* 2001. 3(5): p. 334-7.
[16] Robertson, I., et al., Prospective analysis of stoma-related complications. *Colorectal Dis.* 2005. 7(3): p. 279-85.
[17] Duchesne, J.C., et al., Stoma complications: a multivariate analysis. *Am. Surg.* 2002. 68(11): p. 961-6; discussion 966.
[18] Nastro, P., et al., Complications of intestinal stomas. *Br. J. Surg.* 2010. 97(12): p. 1885-9.
[19] Porter, J.A., et al., Complications of colostomies. *Dis. Colon. Rectum.* 1989. 32(4): p. 299-303.
[20] Feinberg, S.M., R.S. McLeod, and Z. Cohen, Complications of loop ileostomy. *Am. J. Surg.* 1987. 153(1): p. 102-7.
[21] Edwards, D.P., et al., Stoma-related complications are more frequent after transverse colostomy than loop ileostomy: a prospective randomized clinical trial. *Br. J. Surg.* 2001. 88(3): p. 360-3.
[22] Farnham, S.B. and M.S. Cookson, Surgical complications of urinary diversion. *World J. Urol.* 2004. 22(3): p. 157-67.
[23] Fitzgerald, J., et al., Stomal construction, complications, and reconstruction. *Urol. Clin. North Am.* 1997. 24(4): p. 729-33.
[24] Fontaine, E., et al., Twenty-year experience with jejunal conduits. *Urology*, 1997. 50(2): p. 207-13.
[25] Jaffe, B.M., E.M. Bricker, and H.R. Butcher, Jr., Surgical complications of ileal segment urinary diversion. *Ann. Surg.* 1968. 167(3): p. 367-76.
[26] Marshall, F.F., W.F. Leadbetter, and S.P. Dretler, Ileal conduit parastomal hernias. *J. Urol.* 1975. 114(1): p. 40-2.
[27] Guenaga, K.F., ct al., Ileostomy or colostomy for temporary decompression of colorectal anastomosis. *Cochrane Database Syst. Rev.* 2007(1): p. CD004647.
[28] Tilney, H.S., et al., Comparison of outcomes following ileostomy versus colostomy for defunctioning colorectal anastomoses. *World J. Surg.* 2007. 31(5): p. 1142-51.
[29] Allen-Mersh, T.G. and J.P. Thomson, Surgical treatment of colostomy complications. *Br. J. Surg.* 1988. 75(5): p. 416-8.

[30] Scarpa, M., M. Barollo, and M.R. Keighley, Ileostomy for constipation: long-term postoperative outcome. *Colorectal Dis.* 2005. 7(3): p. 224-7.
[31] Williams, J.G., et al., Paraileostomy hernia: a clinical and radiological study. *Br. J. Surg.* 1990. 77(12): p. 1355-7.
[32] Shabbir, J. and D.C. Britton, Stoma Complications: A literature overview. *Colorectal Dis.* 2009.
[33] Janes, A., Y. Cengiz, and L.A. Israelsson, Randomized clinical trial of the use of a prosthetic mesh to prevent parastomal hernia. *Br. J. Surg.* 2004. 91(3): p. 280-2.
[34] Cengiz, Y. and L. Israelsson, Parastomal hernia. *European Surgery*, 2003, 2003. 35: p. 28-31.
[35] Thorlakson, R.H., Technique of Repair of Herniations Associated with Colonic Stomas. *Surg. Gynecol. Obstet.* 1965. 120: p. 347-50.
[36] Etherington, R.J., et al., Demonstration of para-ileostomy herniation using computed tomography. *Clin. Radiol.* 1990. 41(5): p. 333-6.
[37] Cingi, A., et al., Enterostomy site hernias: a clinical and computerized tomographic evaluation. *Dis. Colon. Rectum.* 2006. 49(10): p. 1559-63.
[38] Janes, A., Y. Cengiz, and L.A. Israelsson, Preventing parastomal hernia with a prosthetic mesh. *Arch. Surg.* 2004. 139(12): p. 1356-8.
[39] Arumugam, P.J., et al., A prospective audit of stomas--analysis of risk factors and complications and their management. *Colorectal Dis.* 2003. 5(1): p. 49-52.
[40] Burns, F.J., Complications of colostomy. *Dis. Colon. Rectum.* 1970. 13(6): p. 448-50.
[41] Hulten, L., J. Kewenter, and N.G. Kock, [Complications of ileostomy and colostomy and their treatment]. *Chirurg*, 1976. 47(1): p. 16-21.
[42] Pearl, R.K., et al., A survey of technical considerations in the construction of intestinal stomas. *Am. Surg.* 1985. 51(8): p. 462-5.
[43] Marks, C.G. and J.K. Ritchie, The complications of synchronous combined excision for adenocarcinoma of the rectum at St Mark's Hospital. *Br. J. Surg.* 1975. 62(11): p. 901-5.
[44] Whittaker, M. and J.C. Goligher, A comparison of the results of extraperitoneal and intraperitoneal techniques for construction of terminal iliac colostomies. *Dis. Colon. Rectum.* 1976. 19(4): p. 342-4.
[45] Martin, L. and G. Foster, Parastomal hernia. *Ann. R. Coll. Surg. Engl.* 1996. 78(2): p. 81-4.
[46] Liu, J., et al., Stoma formation for fecal diversion: a plea for the laparoscopic approach. *Tech. Coloproctol.* 2005. 9(1): p. 9-14.

[47] Carne, P.W., et al., Parastomal hernia following minimally invasive stoma formation. *ANZ J. Surg.* 2003. 73(10): p. 843-5.
[48] Sjodahl, R., B. Anderberg, and T. Bolin, Parastomal hernia in relation to site of the abdominal stoma. *Br. J. Surg.* 1988. 75(4): p. 339-41.
[49] Ortiz, H., Does the difference in muscle structure of the rectus abdominis muscle of patients wearing a colostomy or ileostomy explain the different frequency of parastomal hernias? *Int. J. Colorectal Dis.* 1995. 10(1): p. 55.
[50] Pearl, R.K., et al., Early local complications from intestinal stomas. *Arch. Surg.* 1985. 120(10): p. 1145-7.
[51] de Ruiter, P. and A.B. Bijnen, Successful local repair of paracolostomy hernia with a newly developed prosthetic device. *Int. J. Colorectal Dis.* 1992. 7(3): p. 132-4.
[52] Turnbull, R.B., Jr., Intestinal stomas. *Surg. Clin. North Am.* 1958. 38(5): p. 1361-72.
[53] Babcock, G., B.A. Bivins, and C.R. Sachatello, Technical complications of ileostomy. *South Med. J.* 1980. 73(3): p. 329-31.
[54] Nguyen, M.H. and F. Pittas, *How large should a skin trephine be for an end stoma? Aust. N Z J. Surg.* 1999. 69(9): p. 675-6.
[55] Resnick, S., New method of bowel stoma formation. *Am. J. Surg.* 1986. 152(5): p. 545-8.
[56] Rubin, M.S., D.J. Schoetz, Jr., and J.B. Matthews, Parastomal hernia. Is stoma relocation superior to fascial repair? *Arch. Surg.* 1994. 129(4): p. 413-8; discussion 418-9.
[57] Bewes, P.C., Parastomal hernia. *Ann. R. Coll. Surg. Engl.* 1997. 79(2): p. 154-5.
[58] Cheung, M.T., N.H. Chia, and W.Y. Chiu, Surgical treatment of parastomal hernia complicating sigmoid colostomies. *Dis. Colon. Rectum.* 2001. 44(2): p. 266-70.
[59] Horgan, K. and L.E. Hughes, Para-ileostomy hernia: failure of a local repair technique. *Br. J. Surg.* 1986. 73(6): p. 439-40.
[60] Riansuwan, W., et al., Surgery of recurrent parastomal hernia: direct repair or relocation? *Colorectal Dis.* 2010. 12(7): p. 681-6.
[61] Botet, X., E. Boldo, and J.M. Llaurado, Colonic parastomal hernia repair by translocation without formal laparotomy. *Br. J. Surg.* 1996. 83(7): p. 981.
[62] Kaufman, J.J., Repair of parastomal hernia by translocation of the stoma without laparotomy. *J. Urol.* 1983. 129(2): p. 278-9.

[63] Taylor, R.L., Jr., J.L. Rombeau, and R.B. Turnbull, Jr., Transperitoneal relocation of the ileal stoma without formal laparotomy. *Surg. Gynecol. Obstet.* 1978. 146(6): p. 953-8.
[64] Baig, M.K., et al., *Outcome of parastomal hernia repair with and without midline laparotomy.* Tech. Coloproctol. 2006. 10(4): p. 282-6.
[65] Leslie, D., The parastomal hernia. *Surg. Clin. North Am.* 1984. 64(2): p. 407-15.
[66] Cheung, M.T., Complications of an abdominal stoma: an analysis of 322 stomas. *Aust. N Z J. Surg.* 1995. 65(11): p. 808-11.
[67] Moore, T.C. and H. Siderys, The use of pliable plastics in the repair of abdominal wall defects. Ann. *Surg.* 1955. 142(6): p. 973-9.
[68] Kaito, C. and K. Sekimizu, Colony spreading in Staphylococcus aureus. *J. Bacteriol.* 2007. 189(6): p. 2553-7.
[69] Bliziotis, I.A., et al., Mesh-related infection after hernia repair: case report of an emerging type of foreign-body related infection. *Infection*, 2006. 34(1): p. 46-8.
[70] Kercher, K.W., et al., Successful salvage of infected PTFE mesh after ventral hernia repair. *Ostomy Wound Manage*, 2002. 48(10): p. 40-2, 44-5.
[71] Paton, B.L., et al., Management of infections of polytetrafluoroethylene-based mesh. *Surg. Infect. (Larchmt)*, 2007. 8(3): p. 337-41.
[72] Petersen, S., et al., Deep prosthesis infection in incisional hernia repair: predictive factors and clinical outcome. *Eur. J. Surg.* 2001. 167(6): p. 453-7.
[73] Abramov, D., et al., Antibiotic prophylaxis in umbilical and incisional hernia repair: a prospective randomised study. *Eur. J. Surg.* 1996. 162(12): p. 945-8; discussion 949.
[74] Aufenacker, T.J., et al., Systematic review and meta-analysis of the effectiveness of antibiotic prophylaxis in prevention of wound infection after mesh repair of abdominal wall hernia. *Br. J. Surg.* 2006. 93(1): p. 5-10.
[75] Morris-Stiff, G. and L.E. Hughes, The continuing challenge of parastomal hernia: failure of a novel polypropylene mesh repair. *Ann. R. Coll. Surg. Engl.* 1998. 80(3): p. 184-7.
[76] Tekkis, P.P., H.M. Kocher, and J.G. Payne, Parastomal hernia repair: modified thorlakson technique, reinforced by polypropylene mesh. *Dis. Colon. Rectum.* 1999. 42(11): p. 1505-8.
[77] Martínez-Munive, A., et al., Intraparietal mesh repair for parastomal hernias. *Hernia*, 2000. 4: p. 272-274.

[78] Aldridge, A.J. and J.N. Simson, Erosion and perforation of colon by synthetic mesh in a recurrent paracolostomy hernia. *Hernia*, 2001. 5(2): p. 110-2.
[79] Steele, S.R., et al., Is parastomal hernia repair with polypropylene mesh safe? *Am. J. Surg.* 2003. 185(5): p. 436-40.
[80] Abaza, R., P. Perring, and J.J. Sferra, Novel parastomal hernia repair using a modified polypropylene and PTFE mesh. *J. Am. Coll. Surg.* 2005. 201(2): p. 316-7.
[81] Ballas, K.D., et al., Intraperitoneal ePTFE mesh repair of parastomal hernias. *Hernia*, 2006. 10(4): p. 350-3.
[82] Berger, D. and M. Bientzle, Polyvinylidene fluoride: a suitable mesh material for laparoscopic incisional and parastomal hernia repair! A prospective, observational study with 344 patients. *Hernia*, 2009. 13(2): p. 167-72.
[83] Byers, J.M., J.B. Steinberg, and R.G. Postier, *Repair of parastomal hernias using polypropylene mesh*. *Arch. Surg.* 1992. 127(10): p. 1246-7.
[84] de Ruiter, P. and A.B. Bijnen, Ring-reinforced prosthesis for paracolostomy hernia. *Dig. Surg.* 2005. 22(3): p. 152-6.
[85] Greenstein, A.J. and R.A. Aldoroty, Parastomal hernia repair using cross-linked porcine dermis: report of a case. *Surg. Today*, 2008. 38(11): p. 1048-51.
[86] Ripetti, V., et al., First experience for the laparoscopic treatment of parastomal hernia with the use of Parietex composite mesh. *Updates Surg.* 2010.
[87] Rose, J., et al., *Minimal abdominal adhesions after Sepramesh repair of a parastomal hernia*. *Can. J. Surg.* 2009. 52(5): p. E211-2.
[88] Taner, T., et al., *The use of human acellular dermal matrix for parastomal hernia repair in patients with inflammatory bowel disease: a novel technique to repair fascial defects*. *Dis. Colon. Rectum.* 2009. 52(2): p. 349-54.
[89] Franklin, M.E., Jr., et al., The use of porcine small intestinal submucosa as a prosthetic material for laparoscopic hernia repair in infected and potentially contaminated fields: long-term follow-up. *Surg. Endosc.* 2008. 22(9): p. 1941-6.
[90] Rosin, J.D. and R.A. Bonardi, Paracolostomy hernia repair with Marlex mesh: a new technique. *Dis. Colon. Rectum.*, 1977. 20(4): p. 299-302.
[91] Chand, M., et al., Mesh erosion following laparoscopic incisional hernia repair. *Hernia*, 2010.

[92] Sistla, S.C., et al., Enterocutaneous fistula due to mesh fixation in the repair of lateral incisional hernia: a case report. *Cases J.* 2008. 1(1): p. 370.
[93] Seelig, M.H., et al., [Enterocutaneous fistula after Marlex net implantation. A rare complication after incisional hernia repair]. *Chirurg*, 1995. 66(7): p. 739-41.
[94] Hansson, B.M., R.P. Bleichrodt, and I.H. de Hingh, Laparoscopic parastomal hernia repair using a keyhole technique results in a high recurrence rate. *Surg. Endosc.* 2009. 23(7): p. 1456-9.
[95] Berger, D., Prevention of parastomal hernias by prophylactic use of a specially designed intraperitoneal onlay mesh (Dynamesh IPST). *Hernia*, 2008. 12(3): p. 243-6.
[96] Kelly, M.E. and S.W. Behrman, *The safety and efficacy of prosthetic hernia repair in clean-contaminated and contaminated wounds. Am. Surg.* 2002. 68(6): p. 524-8; discussion 528-9.
[97] Geisler, D.J., et al., Safety and outcome of use of nonabsorbable mesh for repair of fascial defects in the presence of open bowel. *Dis. Colon. Rectum.* 2003. 46(8): p. 1118-23.
[98] LeBlanc, K.A., et al., Laparoscopic parastomal hernia repair. *Hernia*, 2005. 9(2): p. 140-4.
[99] Hiles, M., R.D. Record Ritchie, and A.M. Altizer, Are biologic grafts effective for hernia repair?: a systematic review of the literature. *Surg. Innov.* 2009. 16(1): p. 26-37.
[100] Milburn, M.L., et al., Acellular dermal matrix compared with synthetic implant material for repair of ventral hernia in the setting of peri-operative Staphylococcus aureus implant contamination: a rabbit model. *Surg. Infect. (Larchmt)*, 2008. 9(4): p. 433-42.
[101] Kasperk, R., U. Klinge, and V. Schumpelick, The repair of large parastomal hernias using a midline approach and a prosthetic mesh in the sublay position. *Am. J. Surg.* 2000. 179(3): p. 186-8.
[102] Abdu, R.A., Repair of paracolostomy hernias with Marlex mesh. *Dis. Colon. Rectum.* 1982. 25(6): p. 529-31.
[103] Bayer, I., S. Kyzer, and C. Chaimoff, A new approach to primary strengthening of colostomy with Marlex mesh to prevent paracolostomy hernia. *Surg. Gynecol. Obstet.* 1986. 163(6): p. 579-80.
[104] Heniford, B.T., et al., Laparoscopic repair of ventral hernias: nine years' experience with 850 consecutive hernias. *Ann. Surg.* 2003. 238(3): p. 391-9; discussion 399-400.

[105] Hopkins, T.B. and A. Trento, Parastomal ileal loop hernia repair with marlex mesh. *J. Urol.* 1982. 128(4): p. 811-2.
[106] Leslie, D., *The parastomal hernia.* Aust N Z J Surg, 1981. 51(5): p. 485-6.
[107] Alexandre, J.H. and J.L. Bouillot, Paracolostomal hernia: repair with use of a Dacron prosthesis. *World J. Surg.* 1993. 17(5): p. 680-2.
[108] Sugarbaker, P.H., Prosthetic mesh repair of large hernias at the site of colonic stomas. *Surg. Gynecol. Obstet.* 1980. 150(4): p. 576-8.
[109] Stelzner, S., G. Hellmich, and K. Ludwig, Repair of paracolostomy hernias with a prosthetic mesh in the intraperitoneal onlay position: modified Sugarbaker technique. *Dis. Colon. Rectum.* 2004. 47(2): p. 185-91.
[110] van Sprundel, T.C. and A. Gerritsen van der Hoop, Modified technique for parastomal hernia repair in patients with intractable stoma-care problems. *Colorectal. Dis.* 2005. 7(5): p. 445-9.
[111] Bickel, A., E. Shinkarevsky, and A. Eitan, Laparoscopic repair of paracolostomy hernia. *J. Laparoendosc. Adv. Surg. Tech. A*, 1999. 9(4): p. 353-5.
[112] Gould, J.C. and E.C. Ellison, Laparoscopic parastomal hernia repair. *Surg. Laparosc. Endosc. Percutan. Tech.* 2003. 13(1): p. 51-4.
[113] LeBlanc, K.A. and D.E. Bellanger, Laparoscopic repair of paraostomy hernias: early results. *J. Am. Coll. Surg.*, 2002. 194(2): p. 232-9.
[114] Safadi, B., Laparoscopic repair of parastomal hernias: early results. *Surg. Endosc.*, 2004. 18(4): p. 676-80.
[115] Muysoms, E.E., et al., Laparoscopic repair of parastomal hernias: a multicentre retrospective review and shift in technique. *Acta Chir. Belg.*, 2008. 108(4): p. 400-4.
[116] Sugarbaker, P.H., Peritoneal approach to prosthetic mesh repair of paraostomy hernias. *Ann. Surg.*, 1985. 201(3): p. 344-6.
[117] Mancini, G.J., et al., Laparoscopic parastomal hernia repair using a nonslit mesh technique. *Surg. Endosc.*, 2007. 21(9): p. 1487-91.
[118] Porcheron, J., B. Payan, and J.G. Balique, Mesh repair of paracolostomal hernia by laparoscopy. *Surg. Endosc.*, 1998. 12(10): p. 1281.
[119] Voitk, A., Simple technique for laparoscopic paracolostomy hernia repair. *Dis. Colon. Rectum.*, 2000. 43(10): p. 1451-3.
[120] Kozlowski, P.M., P.C. Wang, and H.N. Winfield, Laparoscopic repair of incisional and parastomal hernias after major genitourinary or abdominal surgery. *J. Endourol.*, 2001. 15(2): p. 175-9.
[121] Dunet, F., et al., Laparoscopic management of parastomal hernia in transileal urinary diversion. *J. Urol*, 2002. 167(1): p. 236-7.

[122] Pekmezci, S., et al., Laparoscopic giant parastomal hernia repair with prosthetic mesh. *Tech. Coloproctol.*, 2002. 6(3): p. 187-90.
[123] Deol, Z.K. and V. Shayani, Laparoscopic parastomal hernia repair. *Arch. Surg.*, 2003. 138(2): p. 203-5.
[124] Hansson, B.M., I.H. de Hingh, and R.P. Bleichrodt, Laparoscopic parastomal hernia repair is feasible and safe: early results of a prospective clinical study including 55 consecutive patients. *Surg. Endosc.*, 2007. 21(6): p. 989-93.
[125] Garcia-Vallejo, L., et al., Parastomal hernia repair: laparoscopic ventral hernia meshplasty with stoma relocation. The current state and a clinical case presentation. *Hernia*, 2010.
[126] Marimuthu, K., et al., Prevention of parastomal hernia using preperitoneal mesh: a prospective observational study. *Colorectal. Dis.*, 2006. 8(8): p. 672-5.
[127] Gogenur, I., et al., Prevention of parastomal hernia by placement of a polypropylene mesh at the primary operation. *Dis. Colon. Rectum*, 2006. 49(8): p. 1131-5.
[128] Helgstrand, F., I. Gogenur, and J. Rosenberg, Prevention of parastomal hernia by the placement of a mesh at the primary operation. *Hernia*, 2008. 12(6): p. 577-82.
[129] Light, H.G., A secure end colostomy technique. *Surg. Gynecol. Obstet*, 1992. 174(1): p. 67-8.
[130] Hammond, T.M., et al., Parastomal hernia prevention using a novel collagen implant: a randomised controlled phase 1 study. *Hernia*, 2008. 12(5): p. 475-81.
[131] Serra-Aracil, X., et al., Randomized, controlled, prospective trial of the use of a mesh to prevent parastomal hernia. *Ann. Surg.*, 2009. 249(4): p. 583-7.
[132] Janes, A., Y. Cengiz, and L.A. Israelsson, Preventing parastomal hernia with a prosthetic mesh: a 5-year follow-up of a randomized study. *World J. Surg.*, 2009. 33(1): p. 118-21; discussion 122-3.
[133] Wijeyekoon, S.P., et al., Prevention of parastomal herniation with biologic/composite prosthetic mesh: a systematic review and meta-analysis of randomized controlled trials. *J. Am. Coll. Surg.*, 2010. 211(5): p. 637-45.

In: Hernias: Types, Symptoms and Treatment   ISBN: 978-1-61324-125-7
Editor: James H. Wagner   © 2011 Nova Science Publishers, Inc.

Chapter 3

Hernias:
Types, Symptoms and Treatment

Ho-Hsing Lin and Chi-Wen Juan
Department of Emergency Medicine, Kaosiung Medical University,
Chung-Ho Memorial Hospital, Kaohsiung, Taiwan

Abstract

The Greek term 'hernois' meaning bulge to describe abdominal hernias. The definition of hernia is 'A protrusion of any viscus from its proper cavity. There are abdominal, diaphragmatic, femoral, perineal, lumbar hernia ect. (classified according to the sites).Recognition of the typical appearance of various types of hernia and associated adverse features such as bowel obstruction, strangulation, incarceration, perforation or volvulus formation can help in formulating an accurate diagnosis. It is important to be familiar to hernia for all physicians because it can occur with morbidity and mortality. Thus, early and accurate diagnosis is important.

Abdominal Wall Hernia
(Primary Ventral Hernia)

The hernias are not associated with a fascial scar or related to a trauma. External abdominal hernias are usually detected clinically whereas internal abdominal hernia are usually diagnosed as on imaging or at surgery. Hernia may be detected on radiography, ultra-sonography(US), computed tomography(CT), or magnetic resonance imaging(MRI).

External Abdominal Hernia

Inguinal Hernia

It can be classified into 2 types. In-direct or direct.

It can be classified as reducible or irreducible. Irreducible inguinal hernia can be described as obstructed, incarcerated, gangrenous or non-gangrenous change of intestine according to operative findings.

Indirect inguinal hernias are responsible for almost all inguinal hernia in children. The hernias are more common in men. It is due to patent processus vaginalis.

The locating of the internal ring(deep ring) is between the mid-inguinal point(situated mid-way between the anterior superior iliac spine (ASIS) and the symphisis pubis.

The boundaries:

The arched lower margin of the transversalis fascia (above and laterally
Inferior epigastric vessels (below and medially)

It transmits the spermatic cord in the male, the round ligament in the female.

The inguinal canal is a passage in the anterior abdominal wall. Its direction is oblique interiorly, anteriorly and medially. The contents of the inguinal canal in male are the spermatic cord and the ilio-inguinal nerve; in female are the round ligament of uterus and the ilio-inguinal nerve.

The external inguinal ring (superficial ring)is in anterior wall of the abdomen. It forms the exit of the inguinal canal. It is found within the external oblique aponeurosis, immediately above the pubic crest.

The hernia sac is located lateral to the inferior epigastric vessels.

The incidence of direct inguinal hernia is 25-30% of the inguinal hernia. It enters through a weak point in the fascia of abdominal wall, Hesselbach triangle (rectus abdominis muscle medially, inferior epigastric vessels superior and laterally, inguinal ligament inferiorly).The hernia is more in men and are often bilateral. It is located to inferior epigastric vessels.

The symptom of the inguinal hernia is swelling in the groin which appears on straining, lifting, standing and coughing. It was disappeared when lying. Thus, we have to differentiate the type (indirect and direct); reducible and irreducible. Sometimes, the swelling in groin can not disappear itself and thinks as irreducible. We have to note the time of occurrence ,any associated symptoms, vomiting ,abdominal distension and intensity and duration of pain(obstruction of intestine).The contents of the hernia were greater omentum, small intestine, vermiform appendix(called Amyand's hernia), Meckel's diverticulum(called Littre's hernia).The contents that irreducible inguinal hernia, can be reduced by physician (i.e. the thigh in flexion position and the contents were pushed back to abdominal cavity).If it is reducible, the patient was encouraged for elective operation. Sometimes, it can not be successful. X-ray of abdomen revealed air-fluid level and emergent operation was arranged. Signs of potential strangulation include erythema of the overlying skin, elevated WBC count and fever. On CT, strangulation includes free fluid within the hernia sac, bowel wall thickening, abnormal or lack of mural enhancement, mesenteric haziness and ascites. In advanced cases of strangulation, pneumatosis intestinalis may be present. If, the bowel was gangrenous change, resection and anastomosis (end to end).

Choice of anaesthetics: Local; Spinal; General anaesthesia.

LA: Advantage:

Decrease cardiac, CNS and respiratory complication. Thus, it is suitable for elderly; Low incidence of urine retention;

Visualization of the repair that is complete at operation room (let the patient to strain or coughing);

Absence of post-operative nausea, vomiting, urine retention;

Cost-effective,(economic).

Disadvantage

Pain during operation, thus more/repeat analgesia injection prescribed

SA: Advantage

Not require GA

Required anesthetist and his choice (SA, Epidural Anesthesia)

Disadvantage
On Foley catheter for urinary retention

GA: Advantage
Operation field condition better than LA
Disadvantage
Not suitable for elderly
Urine retention and requires on foley catheterization
Accuracy of repair can not know on the spot

Treatment

Non-operative: used a truss- a device that held a pad firmly against the deep ring.
Operation : Hernia repair (herniorrhaphy)
A single dose of broad-sprectum antibiotics is for high risk patient.
(DM, immune-compromised, elderly)
Bassini repair: High ligation of the hernia sac and reinforcement of the inguinal canal with a three layers closure with interrupted permanent sutures. It is used for direct and indirect hernia.
Marcy repair: It is a simple ring closure, which involves high ligation of hernia sac and obliteration of the deep internal ring with permanent sutures.
Anterior repair: The most common operative approach for inguinal hernias. A transversely oriented, linearly, or slightly curvilinear incision 2 to 3cm above and parallel to the inguinal ligament. Dissected through the subcutaneous tissues,and the Scarpa's fascia. Identification of the external oblique fascia and the external ring are required. The external oblique fascia is incised through the superficial inguinal ring to expose inguinal canal. The neck of sac is ligated at the level of internal ring and excised excess sac. A lipoma of the cord represents retroperitoneal fat that has herniated through the deep inguinal ring and should be suture ligation and removed.
Ilio-pubic tract repair: The transversus abdominis arch to interrupted sutures. It begins at the pubic tubercle and extended laterally past the internal inguinal ring.

Shouldice repair: Multilayer repair. Transversus abdominis aponerurotic arch to ilio-pubic tract. Next, internal oblique and transversus abdominis muscle are sutured to inguinal ligament.

Cooper ligament (McVay) repair: Approximate the edge of transversus abdominis aponeurosis to Cooper's ligament. This repair is the need for relaxing incision. The relaxing incision is made by reflecting the external oblique aponeurosis cephalad and medial to expose the anterior rectus sheath.

Laparoscopic technique: Intra-peritoneal onlay mesh.

The procedure can increase risk of abdominal adhesion.
Trans-abdominal pre-peritoneal prosthetic repair (TAP)
The abdomen is entered laparoscopically and the inguinal peritoneum and the inguinal peritoneum incised requiring closure of the entry point upon completion of the repair. The benefit is low abdominal adhesion.
Totally extra-peritoneal prosthesis repair (TEP)
Placement of the prosthesis (preperitoneally). Balloon insufflation to create a peritoneal space between the peritoneum and transversalis fascial mesh is tracked into place.

The common causes for recurrence after laparoscopic repair are improperly sized and anchored mesh. Common complications following the herniorrhaphy are ecchymosed of penis or scrotum, chronic groin pain (inguinodynia). This emphasizes the importance of recognizing and avoiding the nerve intra-operatively.

Femoral Hernia

It is extremely rare before the age of 20 and peak incidence is during $4^{th}, 5^{th}, 6^{th}$ decade. Inguinal hernia outnumber femoral hernia nearly 15 or 20 to 1, but frequency of strangulation in two types is equal. Female to male ratio is 4:1. It more frequently found on the right side because of the anatomic position of the sigmoid colon, which provide a tamponade effect on left. It presents a lump in groin in inner upper part of thigh (beneath the inguinal ligament and medially to femoral vessels). It may be reducible or irreducible. The diagnosis is based on physical examination and CT imaging. Treatment is surgically repaired.

1. Femoral approach: Cooper's ligament is attached to inguinal ligament to close femoral canal.
2. Inguinal approach: Inguinal ligament is attached to Cooper's ligament.

3. McVay approach: Approximating to transverse aponeuroticofascial layer to the superior pubic ligament or Cooper's ligament.
4. Henry approach (extra-peritoneal): Apposing the inguinal and the pectineal ligament.

Richter's Hernia

It is a type of hernia where only a part of the bowel wall herniated. It is more common in femoral hernias or at the trocar entry site.

Laugier Hernia

It is a femoral hernia through the lacunar ligament.

Narath Hernia

It is secondary to developmental dysplasia of the hip and displacement of the psoas muscle. The subsequent femoral hernia lies behind femoral vessels.

Cloquet Hernia

It is a hernia concealed behind the pectineus fascia.

Obturator Hernia

Incidence: 0.073% of all hernia. Women are affected more often than male because their broader pelvis and larger obturator canal. It is associated with weight loss because of loss of the protective fat in the obturator canal. The canal is about 1-2cm long, 1cm wide. The content of hernia compressed obturator nerve and produced pain and paresthesia of anterior thigh.

Howship-Romberg test: Extension and abduction of thigh produce pain along the medial thigh to the knee.

Hannington-kiff sign: Loss of adductor reflux.

Diagnosis: KUB and CT imaging

If incarceration of bowel loops, the mortality rate as high as 70%.

Treatment: Reduction of the hernia and covered the obturator orifice with placing polypropylence mesh.

Umbilical Hernia

It occurs at the umbilicus (10% of all infants)

Infantile type: Defect is covered with skin, usually reducible. Defect less than 1cm in diameter close spontaneously by 5 years of age.(1)

Adult type: It is acquired by increasing intra-abdominal pressure. Predisposing factors include obesity, multiple pregnancies, liver cirrhosis with ascites and large abdominal tumors.

The hernia is asymptomatic and presents as a bulge at umbilicus.

Hernia smaller than 1.5cm in diameter become incarcerated twice as often as do larger hernia.

Differential diagnosis of neonatal umbilical mass

Umbilical pyogenic granuloma: small, red, moist, velvety mass.

Umbilical polyp: Firm red mass, doesn't resolve after application of silver nitrite.

Patent urachus: Discharge urine from umbilicus

Omphalo-mesenteric duct remnant: Bilious or fecal discharge from umbilicus.

Treatment:

Infantile type: Observation and resolve spontaneously by the time the child reaches 5 years of age. Adult type: Repair as early as possible with using a mesh.

Epigastric Hernia

Hernia of the linea alba occurring between umbilicus and xiphoid. About 20% are multiple. About 80% are located just off the midline (1). Most are small and are made up pre-peritoneal fat with no sac. Larger hernias with peritoneal sac contain omentum, intra-peritoneal organs.

Incidence: 1.6-3.6% of all abdominal wall hernia (2). It is 3 times more common in men.

Symptoms: Small hernia- epigastric pain

Larger reducible hernia- asymptomatic

Larger incarcerated hernia- acutely painful mass; symptoms related to involve organs.

Diagnosis: Physical examination; Ultrasound; CT imaging.

Treatment: Repair- Open approach

Laparoscopic approach: Repair of larger hernia and multiple.

(Advantage: lower complication rate and faster recovery)

Spigelian Hernia

It is through Spigelian fascia which is aponeurotic layer between lateral edge of rectus abdominis muscle medically and semilunar line laterally. Predisposing factors are obesity, multiple pregnancies, rapid weight loss, chronic obstructive lung diseases, prostate enlargement, ascites, trauma, previous surgery.

Incidence: 0.12 to 2.4% of all abdominal wall hernias. Common in $5^{th}, 6^{th}$ decades.
Female to male ratio is about 1.4:1. (3)
The symptom is non-specific or a lateral buldge or mass when standing.
Physical examination: Most are small and covered by external oblique aponeurosis.
It is difficult to palpate a hernia or hernia defect.
Diagnosis: Ultra-sonography; CT imaging
Treatment: Surgically repair (laparotomy)

Lumbar Hernia

It occurs in areas of posterior abdominal wall. It is bounded by 12 rib superiorly, iliac crest inferiorly, erector spinae muscle posteriorly, posterior border of external oblique muscle anteriorly.
There have 2 anatomical spaces.
Inferior lumbar triangle or Petit's triangle: It is defined by latissimus dorsi, free margin of external oblique muscle and iliac crest.
Superior lumbar triangle or Grynfeltt-lesshalt triangle: It lies deep to latissimus dorsi. It is inverted triangle, is defined by 12th rib, quadratus lumbrosum muscle, internal t oblique muscle. The floor is transversalis fascia. 12th intercostals vessels and nerves are found within the triangle. It is the common site of herniation. (4)
Clinical presentation: There is a bulge, increase with coughing.
Strangulation may occur but is uncommon.
Diagnosis: CT imaging
Treatment: Open anterior approach
Laparoscopic approach (trans-abdominal): It requires mobilization of colon and kidney and used mesh coverage.

Supravesical Hernia

It protrudes through supravesical fossa bounded by medial umbilical fold and median umbilical fold. In the fossa, an incarcerated intestinal hernia is a defect in the integrity of the transverse abdominis and fascia transversalis.
It is classified as prevesical, paravesical, intravesical or retrovesical.
The hernias are very rare.
The hernia is associated with signs and symptoms of intestinal obstruction.
Diagnosis: KUB and CT imaging.
Treatment: Repair through infra-umbilical midline laparotomy using mesh.

Perineal Hernia

Protrude through the pelvic daiphgram.
Primary perineal hernia is rare. (5)
It occurs most commonly in older, multi-parous women.
It presents as unilateral bulge in the area of the libia or gluteal or perineal region.
After contents of sac are reduced, defects are repaired with direct suture or with mesh.

Sciatic Hernia

It is through the greater sciatic foramen.
It is asymptomatic or enlarging mass in gluteal area.
It may mimic sciatica with back or leg pain, owing to compression of sciatic nerve.
Treatment: Trans-peritoneal approach(with small bowel obstruction)
Trans-gluteal approach.

Internal Abdominal Hernia

Incidence: 0.2-0.9%. (6)
It is the protrusion of the viscus through a normal or abnormal mesenteric or peritoneal aperture.
Para duodenal hernia is most common. Others are pericecal, transmesenteric, transomental, intersigmoid, supravesical, herniation through the foramen of Winslow.
It is suspected with signs and symptoms of intestinal obstruction particularly in the absence of inflammatory intestinal diseases, external hernia or previous laparotomy.
Para duodenal hernia
Incidence: 50-55% of all internal abdominal hernias.
Approximately 75% on left side and involve the paraduodenal fossa of Landzert.
Male and female ratio: 3:1. (7)
It is located lateral to the 4th segment of duodenum, beneath a peritoneal fold elevated by inferior mesenteric vein and ascending left colic artery. Small bowel loops enter the sac and protrude posteriorly and to the left, essentially herniating into the descending mesocolon and distal portion of the transverse mesocolon.
25% involved on right side, involves the mesentericoparietal fossa of Waldeyer(a defect in the 1st part of the jejunal mesentry). It's orifice is located

behind the superior mesenteric artery and inferior to transverse segment of duodenum. Small bowel herniated into the ascending mesocolon.

Clinical features: Mild GI complaint to acute intestinal obstruction. When compared with left Para duodenal hernia, those on right are usually larger and are more often fixed.

Diagnosis: Barium contrast- The loops may have mass effect, depressing distal transverse colon and indenting posterior wall of the stomach.

CT abdomen (left Para duodenal hernia): Dilated small bowel loops are seen interposed between the pancreas and the duodenum with displacement of inferior mesenteric vein.

Arteriography or laparotomy finding: The inferior mesenteric vein and ascending left colic artery lie in the anterior-medial border of the left Para duodenal hernia.

CT abdomen (right Para duodenal hernia): These obstructed loops may be seen interposed behind the superior mesenteric artery (8). Presence of the encapsulating membrane was noted.

Angiography: Superior mesenteric artery and its ileocolic branch are situated in the anterior wall of the right Para duodenal hernia sac.

Transmesenteric Hernia

Incidence: 8-10% of all internal abdominal hernias.

Occurs through defect in the mesentery of small bowel (in pediatric, prenatal ischemic accidents seems likely) (in adult, the result of trauma or intraperitoneal inflammation).

3 types

1. Transmesocolic type: most common, occurs after laparoscopic Roux-en-Y gastric bypass operation.
2. Transmesenteric type: through a defect in small bowel mesentery. It is more likely to develop volvulus and strangulation or ischaemia.
3. Peterson type: herniation of small bowel behind the Roux loop.

Signs and symptoms of intestinal obstruction: cramp pain, nausea and distension.

Physical examination: Gordian knot of herniated intestine representing a tender abdominal mass.

Diagnosis: Plain X ray abdomen- mechanical small bowel obstruction, central displacement of adjacent colon.

CT abdomen: Clusters of dilated bowel with mesenteric vessels abnormal crowding and engorgement, main mesenteric trunk displacement to right. Location of hernia bowel loop in the right upper quadrant.

Complication: volvulus and ischemia of herniated small bowels.

Transomental Hernia

Incidence: 1-4% of all internal abdominal hernias, usually older than 50 years.

It most occurs in the right side of the greater omentum. Most have a congenital origin but trauma and inflammation may also produce omental perforation.

Herniation of small bowels, cecum, sigmoid colon and presents that of intestinal obstruction. The intestinal loops in herniation through lesser omentum were confined between stomach, liver and pancreas and were crowed in appearances in the lesser sac.

Pericecal Hernia

Incidence: 10-15% internal abdominal hernias

4 types of the peritoneal recesses in pericecal region

(superior ileocecal recess, inferior ileocecal recess, retrocecal recess and paracolic sulci).

Ileal segment herniates through a defect in the mesentery of the cecum and occupies the right paracolic gutter.

Clinically, presents with colic right lower abdominal pain.

Diagnosis: Plain X ray abdomen- unusual relationship of ileum to cecum.

CT abdomen: dilatation of small intestinal loops adjacent to cecum, edematous small bowel located lateral to cecum,

occasionally extending into the right paracolic gutter,

location of hernia bowel loops in right lower quadrant.

Intersigmoid Hernia

Incidence: 4-8% of internal abdominal hernias.

These hernias involve the intersigmoid fossa, a peritoneal pouch located two loops of the sigmoid colon. It is reducible.

3 types:

1. Intersigmoid type- most common
2. Transmesosigmoid type

3. Intramesosigmoid (least common)- lies within the sigmoid mesocolon.

Diagnosis: Barium enema- retrograde filling of small bowel;

sacculated ileal loops occupying left lower quadrant and elevation and displacement of sigmoid colon to the right.

CT abdomen- Rotation of mesentry along with dilated and encapsulated intestinal loops in the pelvis and accompanying strangulation.

Supravesical Hernia

Foramen of Winslow hernia

Incidence: 6-10% of the internal abdominal hernia.

Herniation of the viscera into the lesser sac.

It is located anterior to IVC and posterior to hepatoduodenal ligament, superior to caudate, inferior to duodenum.

Predisposing factor: enlarged foramen of Winslow;

The excessively mobile intestinal loops because a long mesentery.

Patient presents with upper abdominal pain.

Physical examination: localized tenderness and distension in epigastric region.

Plain X ray abdomen: Gas-containing loops of intestine within the lesser sac, medial and posterior to the stomach.

UGI series: displacement of stomach anteriorly and to the left.

The 1st and 2nd portion of duodenum are also displaced to the left.

CT abdomen: presence of bowel posterior to the stomach which is displaced to the left.

Herniated bowel is located posterior to portal vein, CBD and hepatic artery and anterior to IVC.

Retroanastomotic Hernia

Hernias have been most commonly described with Roux-en-Y formation. If the surgery is of antecolic type, the border of the aperture consist of the transverse mesocolon superiorly, ligament of Treitz inferiorly, and the gastro-jejunostomy site and afferent limb of jejunum anteriorly.

The most common herniated loop consists of the efferent jejunal segment.

Symptom was less vomiting because relative lack of fluid and secretion in gastric pouch or Roux limb.

Physical examination: a tender mass in left upper quadrant. Compared with other types, these hernias are less likely to present with strangulation because of large aperture size.

On radiography: collection of dilated loops in left upper quadrant.
Oral contrast enhancement GI series: may reveal abnormal loop posterior and lateral to gastro-jejunostomy.
CT abdomen: Loops fixed in left upper quadrant.

Incisional and Parastomal Hernias

Inscional hernia may occur in 0.5 to 13% patient.

A parastomal hernia is an incisional hernia. It is related to abdominal wall stroma.
When a stroma is formed for whatever reason, a potential site of weakness is created within the abdominal muscle due to the surgical dissection of the muscle to externalize the bowel.

Classification: 4 types

1. Subcutaneous type with a subcutaneous hernia sac.
2. Interstitial type with hernia sac within muscle/aponeurotic layers.
3. Perstomal type with the bowel prolapsing through a circumferential hernia sac enclosing the stoma.
4. Intrastomal in ileostomies with a hernia sac between the intestinal wall and the everted intestinal layer.

Parastomal hernia was defined as the formation of a hernia beside the stoma.

Stoma proplase was defined as eversion of the stroma through the abdominal wall.

Incidence of parastomal hernia: varies between 5% and 52%.

CT scan can be detected than clinical examination.

With stoma brought through the rectus abdminis muscle, a lower rate of parastomal hernia will be encountered than if brought out lateral to the muscle.

Enterostomal opening in the abdominal wall should not be too large, as layers openings may be associated with an increased risk of parastomal herniation. (9)

Risk factors for parastomal hernia formation include wound infection, old age, corticosteroid use, chronic respiratory disorder and malnutrition, sitting of stroma.

Surgical Treatment

Relocation of the stoma into the another quadrant of the abdominal wall. After relocation, the risk of a recurrent parastomal hernia at the new site at least as high as after primary enterostomy and recurrence rate of 24% to 86%. (10)

Relocation should be to the contra-lateral side of abdomen. The stoma should not be relocated into a quadrant on the same side as this seems to be associated as an increased risk of recurrence.

Then, mesh repair of abdominal wall defect at the primary stoma site.

Onlay mesh repair: placed anterior to anterior rectus aponeurosis.

Inlay mesh repair: placed in abdominal wall defect and sutured to wound edges. The technique has largely abandoned because of the high recurrence rates.

Sublay mesh repair: placed dorsal to the rectus muscle and anterior to the posterior rectus sheath. (most advantageous technique and good result).

Intra-peritoneal onlay mesh repair: placed on peritoneum from within abdominal cavity.

Onlay and sublay mesh repairs produce better result.

Prevention following surgery

- Avoid heavy lifting for 3 months post surgery
- Use a support belt or girdle
- Support stoma and abdomen whilst coughing

Diaphragmatic Hernias in Infants

Incidence: 1 in 4000 live-birth. Left side, more common 80%; right side 20%. (11)

1. Posterolateral defect (Foramen of Bochdalek): most common and are associated with greatest complexity and mortality risk.
2. Anterio/retrosternal defect (Foramen of Morgagni)
3. Crural defect (Para-esophageal hernia)
4. Diaphragmatic agenesis

Clinical features:

Neonate presents with respiratory distress, absence or decrease breath sound on affected side.

Present of bowel loops within the thorax can be detected on ultrasound or MRI during 2nd trimester.

Radiological indices obtained from antenatal imaging studies such as polyhydraminos, lung volume, lung/head ratio and positioning of the left lobe of liver(up in the chest or down in the abdominal cavity).

Worse prognosis: Liver up positioning;

Lung/head ratio <1.4 between 22 and 27weeks gestation (12)

CXR: mediastinal shift. In the left side congenital diaphragmatic hernia, gas filled bowel loops and NG tube in the chest. In the right side congenital diaphragmatic hernia, liver herniation may not be suspected on routine.

Presentation: small size- asymptomatic

Delayed presentations are rarely associated with any cardiopulmonary compromise but risk of incarceration.

It is asociated with cardiac, uro-genital, brain or spinal cord defect. Genetic syndrome associated with trisomy 13, 18 and 21; Fryns syndrome; Denys-Drash syndrome; Donnai-Barrow syndrome.(13)

Clinically, pulmonary hypertension presents after a 'honey-moon period' during the 1st 12 to 24 hours of life where the initial stability is replaced by right to left shunting(either through PDA, foramen ovale or other endo-cardial cushion defects)resulting in hypoxia and hypercarbia.

Initial resuscitation: respiratory monitoring; insertion of NG tube; IV assess; O2 application; laboratory investigation; routine imaging; endo-tracheal intubation, high frequency ventilation.

Ventilatory criteria for ECMO cannulation:

- inability to maintain preductal O2 concentration >85%
- peak inspiratory pressure >28cmH2O
- mean airway pressure >15cmH2O
- pressure resistant hypotension

Management of pulmonary hypertension: pulmonary vasodilators such as inhaled nitric oxide, sildenafil (a type 5 phospho-diesterase inhibitor), prostacyclines and bosentan (an endothelin-1 receptor antagonist)

Surgical repair: large congenital diaphragmatic hernia defects require either abdominal wall muscle flap or a synthetic patch.

Lung transplantation: option for life-threatening pulmonary hypoplasia

Congenital diaphragmatic hernia survivors have a high incidence of respiratory (O2 dependence), nutritional (failure to thrive), musculoskeletal, neurodevelopment, GI morbidity.

Bochdalek's Hernia:

It can be diagnosed antenatally on ultrasound.

Common presentation in neonate: with associated acute respiratory distress.

CXR: abnormal bowel gas in the chest with lack of bowel gas in abdomen

Associated with pulmonary hypoplasia

Morgagni's Hernia
Incidence: 3% of all diaphragmatic hernia. It always occurs on right. (14)
The hernia sac, containing omentum, transverse colon.
It is associated with cardiac anomalies and Down's syndrome.

Prognostic Indicator for Congenital Diaphragmatic Hernia
Lung to thorax transverse area ratio (L/T): <0.08 (mortality 100%)
Lung area to head circumference ratio (LHR): <25% of normal (high probability of postnatal mortality)
Extracorporeal membrane oxygenation (ECMO) calculated relative right sided lung volume (RELV): <45% non-survivors
Respiratory distress withih 1st 6 hour of birth: higher propensity for having pulmonary hypoplasia and higher mortality rate.

Diaphragmatic Hernias in Adults

Bochdalek's Hernia:
Posterolateral defect (incidence 1:12500 to 1:2200 live birth)
In neonate: 85% left side (15)
In adult: right side more frequently

Morgagni's Hernia
Less common than Bochdalek's hernia

The hernias are anterior and usually right-side(an opening beneath the sternocostal junction term Larrey spaces usually filled with fat and covered by pleura superiorly and peritoneum inferiorly.

In infancy, it is associated with dextrocardia, ventricular septal defect, anomalous pulmonary venous return, chromosome abnormalities such as Turner syndrome, Trisomy 13,18,21. Liver, colon, and small bowel are found in hernia.

In adult, it is not associated congenital abnormities. Omental fat is often the only structure in hernia.

Symptoms: shortness of breath, gastro-esophageal reflux, intermittent nausea, vomiting, non-specific abdominal pain.

The most common contents of diaphragmatic hernia are omentum, colon and stomach.

Complication: strangulation, incarceration, perforation.

CXR: herniated bowel loops with air-fluid levels in hemithorax and elevation of the diaphragm.

CT is used to identify the location of hernia and to determine whether and how much stomach, bowel and mesentery has herniated into the chest.

Treatment: Surgical Repair

Abdominal approach allows for easier reduction of the hernia contents.
Thoracic approach is that it provides easier dissection of the hernia sac off the mediastinal and pleural structures.
For small defects that can be closed primarily.
Prosthetic patches are used to close larger defects.
Traumatic diaphragmatic hernia: 3 phases
Acute phase: start at the time of original trauma and continues until recovery.
Latent phase: patient may or may not be symptomatic.
Obstructive phase: herniated viscus becomes incarcerated potentially leading to ischemia, necrosis or perforation.

Acute Traumatic Diaphragmatic Injury

With penetrating trauma, the resulting diaphragmatic defect is often too small for herniation. However, with time, unrecognized diaphragmatic defect may enlarge and result in subsequent herniation of intraabdominal contents into the chest. Injury occurs more commonly in left hemidiaphragm. The stomach is the organ with the highest rate of involvement in acute hernia (48%) followed by the spleen(26%), the small bowel, large bowel, omentum(13%) (16). Right diaphragmatic hernia, herniation of liver is less frequent.

Diagnosis:
History
Symptoms and signs- external penetrating wound in anterior thoraco-abdominal area (awareness of possible)
-shoulder pain, epigastric pain, vomiting,
Physical examination: (+) of bowel sounds in chest or (-) of breath sound because of compression of the lung by the hernia.
CXR: Pneumo-thorax, hemo-thorax or pulmonary contusion, atelectasis
NG tube in left chest (stomach in chest)
Supradiaphragmatic air-fluid level (bowel and stomach in chest)

Herniation of liver presenting as elevated hemi-diaphragm.
CT (chest): for hemodynamically stable patient
Diagnostic peritoneal lavage: RBC count 1000/mm3
MRI: the diaphragm can be visualized
Treatment: laparotomy and repair of hernia
(herniated organs back to abdomen, closure of diaphragm to avoid recurrence)

Chronic Traumatic Diaphragmatic Hernia

Refer in latent and obstructive phases
Symptoms: may be related to GI tract, respiratory tract
Diagnosis: previous trauma
CXR: (+) of abdominal viscera within the chest, possibly in conjunction with the collar sign which is identified as appearance of focal constriction at the site where viscera transverse the diaphragmatic breach.
Identification of NG within left hemi-thorax .
Right sided traumatic diaphragmatic hernia- diaphragm elevation with mediastinal shift.
CT: (+) of herniated viscera within the thorax
MRI: T1 weighted imaging- differentiate diaphragm from adjacent tissue such as lung or liver and thereby demonstrate diaphragmatic defect, tissue protruding through then.
Operation approach (transabdominal) open and laparotomy being successfully and safely used in management.
Complication of laproscopic approach- pneumo-thorax and its concomittent cardiovascular effects which can be avoided by the placement of a chest tube prior to insufflations of the peritoneal cavity.
Defect greater than 10cm, may be better using open approach.

Trans-Diaphragmatic Intercostals Hernia (TIDH)

It causes the defects, secondary to the forceful tearing of the inter-costal muscles. Consequently, it was causing separation of the ribs. Such weakness can lead to lung herniation, abdominal viscera herniation(in presence of associated diaphragmatic rupture).

Paraesophageal Hernia

The hernia is through diaphragmatic esophageal hiatus.

Type I: sliding hernia -migration of gastro-esophageal junction into posterior mediastinum through hiatus because of laxity of the phreno-esophageal ligament.

Type II: true hernia –the fundus herniated through the hiatus alongside abnormally positioned GEJ by a defect in the phreno-esophageal membrane.

Type III: a combination type I and II

Type IV: hernia displacement of the stomach with other organs such as the colon, spleen, and small bowel into the chest.

Symptoms:

1. Caused by obstruction(dysphagia, epigastric pain, vomiting, postprandial fullness, early satiety)
2. Caused by GE reflux –sign related GERD(heart burn, chronic cough, regurgitation, aspiration)
3. Recurrent pneumonia from aspiration
4. Ion deficiency anemia. If the sliding hiatal hernia is large, it can cause Cameron ulcers, erosions of the stomach folds near the hiatus which cause minor internal bleeding. 5% of people have discovered by endoscopy.

Diagnosis:

CXR - retrocardiac air-fluid levels within the intrathoracic stomach.
CT- provides types and location of hernia.
UGI- information about the position of GEJ.
Endoscopy-
Type I: GEJ and gastric pouch extend above the impression made by the diaphragm crura.
Type II- there is a separate orifice containing protruded stomach adjacent to a normally located GEJ.
Type III- large gastric pouch is seen above the diaphragm with the GEJ entering midway along the side of the pouch.
Manometry can evaluate the peristaltic function of the esophageal body.

Treatment:

Lengthening procedure: mobilization of esophagus or by gastroplasty.

Fundoplication was added to prevent reflux and is referred to as Collis-Nissen.

To impove the strength of the crural repair, surgeons have used prosthetic mesh but it may cause erosion into the esophagus, adhesions, fibrotic stricture and dysphagia.

Abdominal Hernia in Pregnancy

Importance for a clinician to diagnose emergent situations which include incarceration, strangulation and perforation caused by hernia because consultation with a surgeon. Emergency operations are mandatory.

Inguinal Hernia

Incidence: 1 in 1000-3000, 75% in multiparas.

Diagnosis: presence of a reducible or non-reducible groin lump.

Cough impulse: expansile.

Palpation of hernia content, can differentiate a solid structure (omentum, uterine fibrosis) from the intestine (gas sound on pressure)

The distinction between groin hernia and round ligament varicosities is difficult to make clinically because the symptoms and signs are similar.

A clue, round ligament varicosities are in coexistence of lower limbs or labial varicosities (typical 'bag of worm' appearance of small varices) (17)
Inguinal endometriosis is rare.

Femoral Hernia

The hernias are more frequent in recurrent hernia than in primary hernia, it has been suggested that femoral hernia may be overlooked during repair of inguinal hernias.

Umbilical Hernia

It do not close spontaneously. Slow enlargement over a period of years is common and strangulation is much more frequent than in pediatric umbilical hernia.Symptoms depend on incarcerated organ and duration of incarceration.

Post-Operative (Incisional) Hernia

The incidence of post-operative hernia is 3% following cesarean sections (18) and is associated with midline incisions.

Diagnosis:

History (previous operations)

Symptoms and signs (abdominal pain, vomiting, (-/+) of flatus, stool passage)

Clinical examination:(abdominal scars with palpable defect in the abdominal wall and distension). A rare, but serious obstetric situation can present when a gravid uterus herniates into an anterior abdominal wall through an incisional hernia (19) (20). If strangulation of the uterus occurs at or near term, emergency laparatomy cesarean delivery, followed by immediate repair of the hernia is recommended. If the uterus is strangulated early in pregnancy, immediate repair should be undertaken and taken to term.

Parastomal Hernia

It is an incisional hernia related to an abdominal wall stoma.

The diagnosis is more difficult to make in the pregnant population because nausea and vomiting affects up to 80% of pregnant women. (21)

Examination should be performed with the patient in standing and supine position performing a Valsalva maneuver. The hernia appears as a bulge around the stoma. Digital examination enables fascial aperture and parastomal tissue assessment.

Treatment: relief of obstruction by NG suction

Surgical intervention

Diaphragmatic Hernia

It is a defect in diaphragm.

If the defect is in the posterolateral aspect, it is called it of Bochdalek.

If it is in the presternal region, it is called it of Morgagni.

The prevalence is 1 per 2000-5000 live births.(22)

Women may be asymptomatic until pregnancy, when further herniation is caused by increased stress on the diaphragm by repeated vomiting in 1st 1/2 of the pregnancy, a rapidly enlarging uterus in 2nd trimester and Valsalva maneuver during labor.

Recurrent vomiting in the 2nd or 3rd trimester associated with epigastric pain, hematemesis or respiratory symptoms should raise the suspicion of complicated congenital diaphragmatic hernia. With progression, potentially fatal complication could occur such as obstruction, torsion, strangulation or infarction of the herniated viscera.(23)

Hiatus Hernia

Abdominal contents are through the esophageal hiatus of the diaphragm.

It occurs in up to 18% of multi-para and 5% of primipara women.(24)

Type I (sliding hernia) (The commonest type): Widening of the muscular hiatial aperture of the diaphragm, allowing cardia to herniated upward.

Type II (paraesophageal): localized defect in the phrenoesophageal membrane. The gastric fundus forms the leading part of the herniation.

Type III: are mixed type of type I and II.

Diagnosis

CXR: may show retrocardiac air in bowel lumen, air-liquid levels if obstruction is present or only mediastinal shift to the contralateral side due to compression.(The dose of usage X ray in the pregnant is small)

Thoracic ultrasonography

CT scan

Treatment

For asymptomatic patient, recommended cesarean delivery after fetal lung maturity with simultaneous repair.

Symptomatic diaphragmatic hernia should be managed without delay because of the associated high maternal and fetal mortality if left uncorrected.

With sign of visceral strangulation, surgical emergency, immediate operation is indicated, irrespective of fetal mortality.

Conclusion

All above these hernias remain a diagnostic challenge for primary health care physician. Prompt diagnosis and proper treatment is important.

References

[1] Muschaweck U. umbilical and epigastric hernia repair. *Surg. Clin. north Am.* 2003; 83(5):207-26.
[2] Lang B, lau H, lee F: Epigastric hernia and its etiology. *Hernia*, 2002; 6(3):148-50.
[3] Spangen L. Spigelian hernia. *World J. Surg.* 1989;13:573-80.
[4] Goodman EH, Speese *J. Lumbar. hernia. Ann. Surg.* 1916;63(5):548-60.

[5] Presis A, Herbig B, Dorner A. Primary perineal hernia: a case report and review of the literature. *Hernia,* 2006;10(5):430-3.
[6] Meyer MA. Dynamic Radiology of the Abdomen: Normal and Pathologic Anatomy. 4th ed. New York, NY: Springer Verlag,1994.
[7] Mathieu O, Lucjani A. Internal abdominal herniations. *AJR,* 2004;183:397-404.
[8] Khan MA, Lo Ay, Vande maele DM. Paraduodenal hernia. *Am. Surg.* 1998; 64:1218-22.
[9] Goligher Jc. Surgery of the anus, colon and rectum. 5th edition. London: Beillie're Tindall;1984.p.894.
[10] Devlin HB, Kingsnorth A. Parastomal hernia. In: Devlin A, Kingsnorth A, editors. Management of abdominal hernia. 2nd edition. London: Butterworths; 1998:p.157-66.
[11] Hedrick HL, Crombleholme TM. Flake AW. Et al. Right congenital diaphragmatic hernia: prenatal assement and outcome. *J. Pediatr. Surg.* 2004;39(3):319-23.
[12] Hedrick HL, Danzer E, Merchant A, et al. liver position and lung-to-head ratio for prediction of extracorporeal membrane oxygenation and survival in isolated left congenital diaphragmatic hernia, *Am. J. Obstet. Gynecol.* 2007;197(4):422e421-4.
[13] Scott DA. Genetics of congenital diaphragmatic hernia. *Semin. Pediatr. Surg.* 2007;16(2):88-93.
[14] Corner Tp, Clagett OT. Surgical treatment of hernia of the foramen of morgagni. *J. Thorac cardiovasc. Surg.* 1966;52:461-8.
[15] Gale E. Bochdalek hernia prevalence and CT characteristics. *Radiology,* 1985;156:449-52.
[16] Hernia WC, Ferri LE, Fata P.et al. The current status of traumatic diaphragmatic injury: lessons learned from 105 patients over 13years. *Ann. Thorac Surg.* 2008;85(3):1044-8.
[17] Frede TE. Ultrasonic visualization of varicosities in the female genital tract. *J. ultrasound med.* 1984;3:365-369.
[18] A desunkan mi AR, Faleyimu B. Incidence and aetiological factors of incisional hernia in post-caesarean operations in a Nigerian hospital. *J. Obstet Gynaecol.* 2003;23:258-260.
[19] Malhotra M, Sharma JB, Wadhwe L et al. Successful pregnancy outcome after cesarean section in a case of gravid uterus growing in an incisional hernia of the anterior abdominal wall. *Indian J. Med. Sci.* 2003;57:501-503.

[20] Deka D, Banerjee N, Takkar D. Incarcerated pregnanat uterus in an incisional hernia. *Int. J. Gynecol. Obstet.* 2000;70:377-379.
[21] Cunningham GF, MacDonald PC, Gant NF et al. William's Obstetrics, 20th edn. Norwalk: Appleton and Lange, 1997.
[22] Madden MR, Paull DE, Finkelstein JL et al. Occult diaphragmatic injury from stab wounds to the lower chest and abdomen. *J. Trauma,* 1989;29:292-298.
[23] Fleyfel M, Provost N, Ferreira JF et al. Management of diaphragmatic hernia during pregnancy. *Anesth. Analg.* 1998;86:501-503.
[24] Rigler LG, Eneboe JB. Incidence of hiatus hernia in pregnant women and its significance. *J. Thorac Surg.* 1935;4:262-266.

In: Hernias: Types, Symptoms and Treatment
Editor: James H. Wagner

ISBN: 978-1-61324-125-7
© 2011 Nova Science Publishers, Inc.

Chapter 4

Impact of Prophylactic Fundoplication on Survival without Growth Disorder in Left Congenital Diaphragmatic Hernias Requiring a Patch Repair

Anne Dariel[1], Jean-Christophe Rozé[2], Hugues Piloquet[3], G. Podevin[1] and the French CDH Study Group

[1]Department of Pediatric Surgery
[2]Neonatal Intensive Care Unit
[3]Department of Pediatrics, University Hospital, Nantes, France

Abstract

Introduction: Congenital diaphragmatic hernia (CDH) requiring a patch repair is likely to develop a more severe gastroesophageal reflux (GER) needing fundoplication during the first months of life. Our hypothesis asserts that a prophylactic fundoplication performed during initial diaphragmatic repair can limit nutritional morbidity. The aim of this retrospective multicenter study was to clarify the relationship between prophylactic fundoplication and survival without growth disorder. Patients and methods: Between 1994 and 2005, 57 cases of left-side congenital diaphragmatic hernia requiring a patch repair were treated in 8 French pediatric surgery units. Prophylactic fundoplication was performed in 34 cases during initial diaphragmatic repair. Forty-three patients survived. Weight-for-height (W/H) and height-for-age (H/A) Z-scores were compared at 3 months, 3 and 5 years between the prophylactic fundoplication group (n=29) and the control group (n=14). The propensity score method was used to limit bias to determine if prophylactic fundoplication was an independent factor of survival without growth disorder (growth disorder was defined by weight-for-height and height-for-age Z-scores <-1.5 SD). Median follow-up was 4,88 years. Results: At 3 and 5 years, H/A Z-scores were significantly higher in prophylactic fundoplication group, -0.35 SD versus -1.19 SD (p=0.02) and -0.26 SD versus -1.31 SD (p=0.002). W/H Z-scores were not statistically different, -1.24 SD versus -1.62 SD (p>0.05) and -1.13 versus -1.4 SD (p>0.05). There was no significant difference between H/A and W/H Z-scores at 3 months or the need and the duration of gastric-tube feeding in the 2 groups. After adjustment for the propensity score, prophylactic fundoplication was significantly associated with survival without growth disorder (p=0.002). Conclusion: In this multicenter study concerning a high-risk population of congenital diaphragmatic hernia requiring a patch repair, we observed a significant relationship between prophylactic fundoplication and survival without growth disorder after adjustment for the propensity score, suggesting that prophylactic fundoplication could prevents growth disorder. Furthermore, it was very interesting to note that prophylactic fundoplication only improved statural growth in these patients. These results must be confirmed by a prospective randomized study and a more detailed growth evaluation would be necessary to explain their unusual growth favouring height over weight.

Introduction

Congenital diaphragmatic hernia (CDH) requiring a patch repair concerns 28 to 44% of CDH and represents a challenge for medical-surgical teams [1-7]. In these severe forms of CDH, survival rate is mainly determined by the high incidence of pulmonary hypoplasia and pulmonary hypertension in the neonatal period. Nutritional morbidity becomes one of the major concerns for survivors and is mainly caused by the development of a severe gastroesophageal reflux (GER), which may worsen an already compromised respiratory status [3-7,10,12,14-15].

GER is reported in up to 60% of cases and frequently requires fundoplication during the first months of life. Patch repair is now well-recognized as a predictor factor of severe GER with failure of medical treatment and need for fundoplication [3,7]. We hypothesized that a prophylactic fundoplication performed during the initial diaphragmatic repair in the neonatal period can limit nutritional morbidity.

1. Patients and Methods

1.1. Patients

Between December 1994 and june 2005, 77 newborn with CDH requiring a patch repair were treated in 8 french units of pediatric surgery. Patients with severe prematurity (gestational age <32 weeks, n=3), low birth weight (<1500g, n=1) and right-side CDH (n=16) were excluded from our study.

Fifty-seven neonates with left-side CDH requiring a patch repair were finally included retrospectively. The indication of patch repair was impossible direct closure without tension because of diaphragmatic aplasia (n=20) or severe hypoplasia (n=37).

Surgery was performed after hemodynamic and respiratory stabilization using « gentle ventilation » and permissive hypercapnia. High-frequency oscillatory ventilation (HFO), inhaled nitric oxide (NO) and extracorporeal membrane oxygenation (ECMO) were used when needed.

1.2. Nutritional Evaluation

Nutritional morbidity was compared for the 43 survivors divided into 2 groups: 29 patients with prophylactic fundoplication and 14 patients without prophylactic fundoplication (control group).

To detect growth disorders, each patient's growth was assessed by his weight-for height (W/H) and height-for-age (H/A) indicators, calculated according to the child growth charts and tables from the World Health Organization, at each 3 months during the first year of life and then at 18 months, 24 months, 3 years and 5 years old.

In order to evaluate growth failure, W/H and H/A « Z-scores » were calculated [16]. Growth disorder was defined by W/H or H/A Z-scores < -1.5 standard deviations (SD), because a -2 SD threshold would have eliminated too many cases and -1 SD would not have been discriminatory. For premature children, we used corrected age.

1.3. Statistical Analysis

Because this study was multicentric and retrospective, we used the propensity score method to reduce bias [17]. The propensity score was defined as a conditional probability between 0 and 1 that the patient will receive the treatment, the prophylactic fundoplication, on the basis of an observed group of covariates. The score is then used as if it was the only confounding covariate to collapse the different covariates between the groups.

A logistic regression model was developed to determine the propensity score for prophylactic fundoplication and included the covariates indicated in Table 1. The 8 centers were divided into 3 groups for the statistical analysis: centers 1 and 2 which had treated more than 15 CDH requiring a patch repair, and the 6 other centers with less than 15 cases each. Three logistic regression models were used to estimate adjusted odds ratios, with 95% confidence intervals, of survival, survival without growth disorder, and survival without growth disorder and delayed fundoplication (performed during a second surgical time for gastroesophageal reflux disease) : (1) no adjustment, (2) adjustment for centers and (3) adjustment for propensity score.

All analysis were performed with SPSS 15.0 (SPSS, Chicago, Illinois). Continuous values were expressed as medians (range values). The Mann-Whitney U test and the χ^2 test were used to compare population characteristics.

2. Results

2.1. Population Characteristics

The pediatric surgeon decided himself to perform or not a fundoplication during the primary diaphragmatic repair on anatomic criteria because of the lack of pre-existent consensus.

Prophylactic fundoplication was performed in 34 patients : complete fundoplication described by Nissen in 14 and partial fundoplication in 20 (Toupet procedure and ventral semi-valve) according to surgical habits and anatomic presentations. The others 20 patients without prophylactic fundoplication were included in the control group.

Table 1. Associations between variables included in the calculation of propensity score and prophylactic fundoplication

Covariates	Infants with prophylactic fundoplication (n=34)	Infants without prophylactic fundoplication (n=23)	aOR	95% CI	P value
Male	18 (52.9%)	16 (69.6%)	1.0	(0.2-4.1)	0.991
Birth weight (<2500g)	2 (5.9%)	4 (17.4%)	0.1	(0.0-1.0)	0.051
Centers					
Others centers	11 (32.4%)	14 (60.9%)	1		
Center 1	11 (32.4%)	6 (26.1%)	2.5	(0.4-16.7)	0.331
Center 2	12 (35.3%)	3 (13.0%)	11.3	(1.6-79.1)	0.015
Age at surgery (day)	5 [2-10]	4 [2-6]	1.3	(1.0-1.7)	0.061
Intrathoracic liver	18 (52.9%)	14 (60.9%)	1.0	(0.1-11.8)	0.992
Associated malformations	8 (23.5%)	9 (39.1%)	0.2	(0.0-1.3)	0.101
Preoperative ECMO	7 (20.6%)	4 (17.4%)	1.8	(0.2-15.6)	0.574

aOR: Adjusted odds ratio
Data are presented as n (%) or median [interquartile]

No complications specifically related to prophylactic fundoplication were noted, but fundoplication was redone during the follow-up in 4. We compared characteristics between the 2 groups with or without prophylactic fundoplication (Table 2). There was no significant difference for prenatal diagnosis, perinatal parameters (sex, age of gestation, birth weight, Apgar), intensive care data (NO, HFO, ECMO), age at primary diaphragmatic repair, intrathoracic liver, associated malformations, follow-up.

Nevertheless prophylactic fundoplication tended to be performed preferentially in centers 1 and 2 that treated more infants with CDH requiring a patch repair (p=0.07). Parenteral nutrition was used in all 57 patients with no significant difference in duration: 37 [11;105] and 36 [9;145] days (p=0.73) in patients with or without prophylactic fundoplication. A gastric tube or gastrostomy was added in 14 and 10 cases respectively (p=0.85) with no significant difference in duration, 27 [4;61] months and 21 [6;48] months respectively (p=0.96). No gastrostomy was performed during initial diaphragmatic repair. For the 23 patients without prophylactic fundoplication, delayed fundoplication was needed in 9 and performed at a median age of 3.25 [2;8] months. Median follow-up was 5.0 [2.0;12.5] and 4.3 [3.0;7.2] years respectively (p=0.45).

Table 2. Comparison of caracteristics between infants with and without prophylactic fundoplication

Caracteristic	Infants with prophylactic fundoplication (n=34)	Infants without prophylactic fundoplication (n=23)	P value
Prenatal diagnosis	33 (97%)	22 (97%)	0.85
Gestational age at prenatal diagnosis (week)	23 [14-32]	23 [16-38.5]	0.17
Male	18 (53%)	16 (70%)	0.25
Birth weight (g)	3000 [2300-3960]	3005 [1890-3800]	0.92
Gestational age at birth (week)	38.3 [34-41.7]	38.1 [34-40]	0.85
Apgar at 1 minute	6 [2-10]	5 [1-10]	0.44
Apgar at 5 minutes	7 [4-10]	6 [3-9]	0.29
Preoperative NO	33 (97%)	22 (97%)	0.85
Preoperative HFO	34 (100%)	23 (100%)	1.00
Preoperative ECMO	9 (26%)	3 (13%)	0.25
Age at primary repair (day)	5 [1-17]	4 [1-13]	0.44
Intrathoracic liver	16 (47%)	9 (39%)	0.60
Associated malformations	8 (24%)	8 (35%)	0.35
Treatment in centers 1 or 2	23 (68%)	10 (43%)	0.07
Follow-up (year)	5.0 [1-12.5]	4.3 [3-7.2]	0.23

Data are presented as n (%) or median [interquartile]

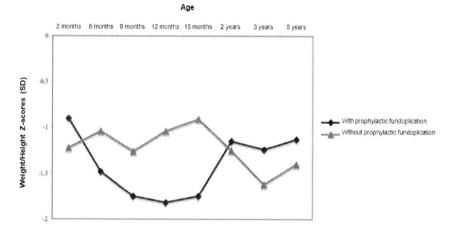

Figure 1. Longitudinal evolution of Weight/Height Z-scores between 3 months and 5 years of follow-up in infanys with and without prophylactic fundoplication.

Table 3. Comparison of W/H and H/A Z-scores between infants with and without prophylactic fundoplication

Follow-up	3 months	6 months	9 months	12 months	18 months	24 months	3 years	5 years
Patients (n)	35	32	32	31	32	32	32	27
W/H Z-score (SD)								
With prophylactic fundoplication	-0.9	-1.48	-1.75	-1.82	-1.75	-1.15	-1.24	-1.13
Without prophylactic fundoplication	-1.22	-1.04	-1.26	-1.04	-0.91	-1.25	-1.62	-1.4
H/A Z-score (SD)								
With prophylactic fundoplication	-1.21	-1.13	-1.07	-0.98	-0.74	-0.72	-0.35*	-0.26**
Without prophylactic fundoplication	-1.33	-1.87	-1.92	-1.38	-1.18	-1.18	-1.19*	-1.31**

* p=0.02, ** p=0.002

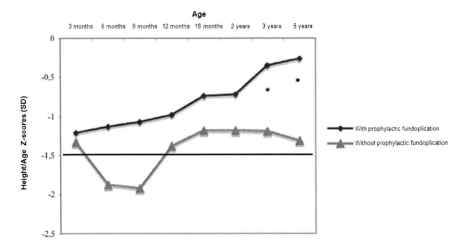

Figure 2. Longitudinal evolution of Height/Age Z-scores between 3 months and 5 years of follow-up in infanys with and without prophylactic fundoplication (* p<0.05).

2.2. Nutritional Evaluation

Nutritional evaluation was possible for the 43 survival infants, 29 with and 14 without prophylactic fundoplication (p=0.04).

2.2.1. W/H Z-Scores (Figure 1, Table 3)

Longitudinal evolution of W/H Z-scores between 3 months and 5 years was not different with or without prophylactic fundoplication, respectively -0.6 DS [-2.27; +2.58] versus -0.4 DS [-3.45;+1.68] (p=0.97). Medians of W/H Z-scores were not different at 3 months, 3 years and 5 years (p>0.05).

2.2.2. H/A Z-Scores (Figure 2, Table 3)

Improvement of H/A Z-scores between 3 months and 5 years tended to be higher with prophylactic fundoplication than without prophylactic fundoplication, respectively +1.22 DS [-0.68;+3.48] versus +0.34 DS [-1.81;+1.4] (p=0.055). At 3 years and 5 years, medians of H/A Z-scores were higher with prophylactic fundoplication, respectively -0.35 DS [-2.33;+1.29] versus -1.19 DS [-2.91;+0.73] (p=0.02) and -0.26 DS [-1.76;+1.02] versus -1.31 DS [-3.24;-0.21] (p=0.002). Medians of H/A Z-scores were not statistically different at 3 months (p=0.71).

2.2.3. Growth Disorders

Growth failure was present in 4/26 and 3/13 infants measured at 6 months (p=0.36), 1/26 and 5/13 at 1 year (p=0.02) and 9/29 and 11/14 (p=0.04) at least once during follow-up, respectively in patients with and without prophylactic fundoplication. Overall, 20/34 and 5/23 survived without growth disorder at the end of follow-up (p= 0.02).

Table 4. Comparison of Z-scores below -1.5 SD at 3 years between infants with and without prophylactic fundoplication

	Z-score <-1.5 SD	P value
W/H		0.6
With prophylactic fundoplication (n=22)	8 (36%)	
Without prophylactic fundoplication (n=10)	5 (50%)	
H/A		0.04
With prophylactic fundoplication (n=22)	2 (9%)	
Without prophylactic fundoplication (n=10)	4 (40%)	

Data are presented as n (%)

Furthermore, at 3 years, H/A Z-scores below -1.5 SD were statistically less frequent with prophylactic fundoplication than without prophylactic fundoplication, respectively 2/22 (9%) children versus 4/10 (40%) (p=0.04). Conversely, W/H Zcores were below -1.5 SD respectively in 8/22 (36%) versus 5/10 (50%), without significant difference (p=0.6) (Table 4).

2.3. Survival and Propensity Score

2.3.1. Propensity Score (Table 1)

The propensity score was calculated for 56 of the 57 newborns included in the study using different covariates that could have influenced the probability of performing prophylactic fundoplication. The choice of fundoplication was not influenced by sex, intrathoracic liver, age at surgery, associated malformations, pre-operative ECMO. Only centers (center 2) and birth weight over 2500g significantly increased or tended to increase the probablility of undergoing prophylactic fundoplication.

2.3.2. Association between Prophylactic Fundoplication and Survival

Fourteen patients died, 5 (15%) with and 9 (39%) without prophylactic fundoplication. Median age at death was 30 [10;214] and 27 [3;457] days (p=0.29), respectively.

Table 5. Association between prophylactic fundoplication and survival without growth disorders, and survival without growth disorders and delayed fundoplication

	OR	95% CI	p value
Survival without growth disorders			
No adjustment	4.0	(1.3-12.8)	0.018
Adjustment for center	5.6	(1.6-20.6)	0.009
Adjustment for propensity score	4.7	(1.2-18.5)	0.028
Survival without growth disorders and delayed fundoplication			
No adjustment	9.5	(2.4-38.3)	0.002
Adjustment for center	13.1	(2.9-60.6)	0.001
Adjustment for propensity score	15.9	(2.8-88.3)	0.002

OR: Odds ratio

Eight patients died before 1 month because of severe pulmonary hypoplasia, 3 with and 5 without prophylactic fundoplication. Six patients died later because of worsening of pulmonary hypertension; growth disorders were present in 1 of the 2 cases with prophylactic fundoplication and in 3 of the 4 cases without prophylactic fundoplication.

Survival per se was not significantly associated with prophylactic fundoplication after adjustment for propensity score (OR 1,4; 95% CI 0,3-0,7; p=0,70). But prophylactic fundoplication was significantly associated with survival without growth disorders and survival without growth disorders and delayed fundoplication (Table 5).

3. Discussion

In this multicenter retrospective study, performing prophylactic fundoplication during initial diaphragmatic repair in left-side CDH requiring a patch repair is positively associated with survival without growth disorders, and survival without growth disorders and delayed fundoplication after adjustment with propensity score. The propensity score method limits recruitment bias and is a way of asserting that the effect of a treatment is compared only between patients who are equally likely to receive it.

GER is a well-known complication in survivors of CDH reported in 30% to 81% of cases and is responsible for an increase of growth disorders and oral aversion [3,10-14]. Physiopathology of GER is not well understood and several mechanisms have been proposed to explain it : (1) abnormalities of the gastroesophageal junction with weakened crura, disruption of angle of Hiss, a shortened abdominal esophagus [18,19], (2) antenatal obstruction of gastroesophageal junction by herniated viscera resulting in esophageal ectasia and esophageal dysmotricity in long-term [13,20], (3) pulmonary hypoplasia causing excessive negative intrathoracic pressure and reintegration of herniated viscera into abdominal cavity increasing the positive intraabdominal pressure [21,22].

Antireflux surgery is needed in 12% to 29% of CDH [3-7,10,12,14-15]. Koivusalo et al demonstrated that the incidence of GER was maximal during the first year after primary diaphragmatic repair and that fundoplication was performed in 15% of cases most commonly before six months of life [4]. Diamond et al confirmed this result with 12% of patients who underwent antireflux surgery at a median age of 4.7 months [5]. Several published studies showed that patients with CDH requiring a patch repair are likely to have development of severe GER needing fundoplication. In Muratore's study, 68% of fundoplications were associated with CDH requiring a patch repair [7]. For Su et al, infants with CDH defects necessitating a patch repair are also likely to develop severe GER (RR=2.31) requiring fundoplication (RR=7.78) [3].

Efficiency of fundoplication is well-established in literature with a wrap integrity found in 86.6% to 98% of cases at long term [23-30], reaching to 93% to 98% in patients without comorbidities and decreasing to 64% to 92.6% in infants with neurologic impairments, chronic respiratory diseases or esophageal congenital malformations. For several authors early fundoplication performed during the first year of life is a predicting factor of GER recurrence (11.1-32%) [31-33]. Redo surgery are classically due to transdiaphragmatic migration of the wrap [25-26], prevented by crura closure and wrap attachment to the crus, or wrap dehiscence secondary to surgical difficulties due to anatomic abnormalities (little stomach, short abdominal portion of esophagus) [6,26]. Literature is really poor concerning fundoplicature efficiency in CDH. Tovar et al demonstrated a wrap integrity in 77% of cases [34]. Only one study was published about prophylactic fundoplication in CDH and showed the efficient decrease of GER incidence from 52.6% to 17.6% [6]. Nevertheless there is no data concerning CDH with patch repair. In our cohort GER was decreased in left-side CDH requiring a patch repair from 89% to 38% with prophylactic fundoplication (data not shown) with no additional surgical risk. The higher recurrency of GER in our study is probably due to anatomic abnormality of the left diaphragmatic crus that makes impossible the crura closure.

GER-related complications are really common in the CDH population such as esophagitis, failure to thrive, growth disorders and recurrent aspirations.

Nutritional morbidity is a chronic concern in the long-term follow-up of CDH requiring a patch repair. A severe pulmonary hypoplasia is often associated and responsible for chronic restrictive respiratory failure [9]. The corresponding lung function impairment results in augmented work of breathing. An increased oxygen cost for respiratory muscles during rest and exercise as well and their impact on malnutrition have often been emphasized in adults chronic respiratory diseases resulting in an imbalance between energy intake and expenditure [35-36]. GER may worsen an already compromised nutritional status with dysphagia and prolonged oral aversion. Growth retardation is common in the CDH population [37-40]. Despite aggressive nutritional management, 56% of infants remained below the 25th percentile for weight in Muratore's report [7], 40% had a weight below the fifth percentile at 1 year after surgery as reported by Lund et al [40], and 21% had a reduced weight-for-height ratio at 2 years in Van Meurs' study [38]. In severe left-side CDH with intrathoracic liver, Cortes et al showed 56% and 22% of weight-for-age ratios below -2 SD at 1 and 2 years [41]. Before our study, the potential benefit of prophylactic fundoplication had not been evaluated, except in neonates with congenital heart diseases: early fundoplication significantly increased long-term weight gain [42]. In our report, prophylactic fundoplication improved height gain with height-for-age ratios significantly higher at 3 and 5 years, but was not efficient for weight gain in CDH requiring a patch repair, reflecting a fragile nutritional balance. This is an unusual growth evolution favouring height over weight that was still described by Muratore et al [7]. A nutritional evaluation would be required to explain their unusual growth.

Assessment of fat-free mass and fat mass would be interesting to perform objective body composition measurements. Anthropometry provides the single most simple, universally applicable, inexpensive and non-invasive technique for assessing the body composition by measuring peripheral muscle strength. Bioelectrical impedance analysis is an objective and also non-invasive method (validated in paediatrics) used in addition to anthropometry in specialized nutrition units [36,43-45]. Infants with severe CDH requiring a patch repair may favour the development of fat-free mass over fat mass to increase muscular mass, and particularly respiratory muscles, to combat chronic respiratory failure.

Respiratory morbidity of GER has never been demonstrated in CDH. We know that patch repair is a predictive factor of severe respiratory failure due to associated pulmonary hypoplasia [8-9,46-47]. GER disease may also deteriorate an already affected respiratory function. Relation between GER and pulmonary symptoms has been studied in children with chronic respiratory diseases as asthma or cystic fibrosis [48]. GER is a well-known factor of aggravation of asthma in children. Two physiopathological mechanisms leading to respiratory symptoms have been demonstrated in GER : chronic pulmonary aspirations and esophageal acid induced-bronchoconstriction. Chronic pulmonary aspirations, represented by the recurrent passage of gastric contents into the subglottic airways, due to proximal GER may result in recurrent pneumoniae, progressive lung disease and bronchectasies [49-50]. A high prevalence of respiratory tract infections has been showed in children with CDH (24-50%), and particularly the first year of life [37]. Esophageal acid induced-bronchoconstriction is related to distal GER and is mediated by esophagobronchial vagal reflex without any aspirations of gastric contents in airways [51]. One explanation of this esophagobronchial vagal reflex is the same embryologic origin of esophagus and inferior airways. The recent development of multiple intraesophageal impedance monitoring in combination with pH measurement allows to distinguish between acid and non-acid esophageal reflux, and to establish the relation between GER and pulmonary symptoms in chronic respiratory diseases [52], that was impossible with the 24-hours esophageal pH testing alone [53]. Field et al suggest in a review of litterature that medical anti-reflux therapy improves asthma symptoms due to distal GER in 69% of cases and reduces asthma medication but has a minimal effect on lung function [54]. In pulmonary symptoms secondary to recurrent aspirations, medical therapy is inefficient and anti-reflux surgery remains the gold-standard with pulmonary symptoms resolution in 48% to 92% of cases [49,55-57]. Respiratory symptoms related to GER decreased or resolved respectively in 76% and 24% of children aged less than 12 months who underwent antireflux surgery for Mattioli et al [58]. Pulmonary morbidity was not studied in our report because of the lack of available retrospective data. Comparison of pulmonary symptoms and respiratory function (lung ventilation and perfusion scintigraphy and/or spirometry) between patients who undergo or not prophylactic fundoplication would be interesting to define if prophylactic fundoplication could protect respiratory function in severe CDH requiring a patch repair.

Conclusion

The retrospective nature of this study is a limiting factor. Nevertheless when we adjusted the propensity score, we adjusted 7 covariates to reflect a center's practice, including nutritional support practice. So the observed association seems to be not biased, although it should be confirmed by a randomized prospective study. We suggest that prophylactic fundoplication can prevent growth disorders in infants with left congenital diaphragmatic hernia requiring a patch repair.

References

[1] Peetsold, MG; Heij, HA. The long-term follow-up of patients with a congenital diaphragmatic hernia: a broad spectrum of morbidity. *Pediatr. Surg. Int.* 2009, 25, 1-17.

[2] Hayward, MJ; Kharasch, V. Predicting inadequate long-term lung development in children with congenital diaphragmatic hernia: an analysis of longitudinal changes in ventilation and perfusion. *J. Pediatr. Surg.* 2007, 42, 112-6.

[3] Su, W; Berry, M. Predictors of gastroesophageal reflux in neonates with congenital diaphragmatic hernia. *J. Pediatr. Surg.* 2007, 42, 1639-43.

[4] Koivusalo, AI; Pakarinen, MP. The cumulative incidence of significant gastroesophageal reflux in patients with congenital diaphragmatic hernia- a systematic clinical, pH-metric and endoscopic follow-up study. *J. Pediatr. Surg.* 2008, 43, 279-82.

[5] Diamond, IR; Mah, K. Predicting the need for fundoplicature at the time of congenital diaphragmatic hernia repair. *J. Pediatr. Surg.* 2007, 42, 1066-70.

[6] Chamond, C; Morineau, M. Preventive antireflux surgery in patients with congenital diaphragmatic hernia. *World J. Surg.* 2008, 32, 2454-8.
[7] Muratore, CS; Utter, S. Nutritional morbidity in survivors of congenital diaphragmatic hernia. *J. Pediatr. Surg.* 2001, 36, 1171-6.
[8] Koumbourlis, AC; Wung, JT. Lung function in infants after repair of congenital diaphragmatic hernia. *J. Pediatr. Surg.* 2006, 41, 1716-21.
[9] Muratore, CS; Kharasch, V. Pulmonary morbidity in 100 survivors of congenital diaphragmatic hernia monitored in a multidisciplinary clinic. *J. Pediatr. Surg.* 2001, 36, 133-40.
[10] Fasching, G; Huber, A. Gastroesophageal reflux and diaphragmatic motility after repair of congenital diaphragmatic hernia. *Eur. J. Pediatr. Surg.* 2000, 10, 360-4.
[11] Koot, VC; Bergmeijer, JH. Incidence and management of gastroesophageal reflux after repair of congenital diaphragmatic hernia. *J. Pediatr. Surg.* 1993, 28, 48-52.
[12] Kieffer, J; Sapin, E. Gastroesophageal reflux after repair of congenital diaphragmatic hernia. *J. Pediatr. Surg.* 1995, 30, 1330-3.
[13] Stolar, CJ; Levy, JP. Anatomic and functional abnormalities of the esophagus in infants surviving congenital diaphragmatic hernia. *Am. J. Surg.* 1990, 159, 204-7.
[14] D'Agostino, JA; Bernbaum, JC. Outcome of infants with congenital diaphragmatic hernia requiring extracorporeal membrane oxygenation: the first year. *J. Pediatr. Surg.* 1995, 30, 10-5.
[15] Lund, DP; Mitchell, J. Congenital diaphragmatic hernia: the hidden morbidity. *J. Pediatr. Surg.* 1994, 29, 258-62.
[16] Waterlow, JC. Note on the assessment and classification of protein energy malnutrition in children. *Lancet,* 1973, 2, 87-9.
[17] Rozé, JC; Denizot, S. Prolonged sedation and/or analgesia and 5-year neurodevelopment outcome in very preterm infants. *Arch. Pediatr. Adolesc. Med.* 2008, 162, 728-33.
[18] Sigalet, DL; Nguyen, LT. Gastroesophageal reflux associated with large diaphragmatic hernias. *J. Pediatr. Surg.* 1994, 29, 1262-5.
[19] Nagaya, M; Akatsuka, H. Gastroesophageal reflux occurring after repair of congenital diaphragmatic hernia. *J. Pediatr. Surg.* 1994, 29, 1447-51.
[20] Stolar, CJ; Berdon, WE. Esophageal dilatation and reflux in neonates supported by ECMO after diaphragmatic hernia repair. *Am. J. Roentgenol.* 1988, 151, 135-7.

[21] Qi, B; Soto, C. An experimental study on the pathogenesis of gastroesophageal reflux after repair of diaphragmatic hernia. *J. Pediatr. Surg.* 1997, 32, 1310-3.

[22] Wang, W; Tovar, JA. Airway obstruction and gastroesophageal reflux: an experimental study on the pathogenesis of this association. *J. Pediatr. Surg.* 1993, 28, 995-8.

[23] Fonkalsrud, EW; Ashcraft, KW. Surgical treatment of gastroesophageal reflux in children: a combined hospital study of 7467 patients. *Pediatrics*, 1998, 101, 467-8.

[24] Taylor, LA; Weiner, T. Chronic lung disease is the leading risk factor correlating with the failure (wrap disruption) of antireflux procedures in children. *J. Pediatr. Surg.* 1994, 29, 161-4.

[25] Ngerncham, M; Barnhart, DC. Risk factors for recurrent gastroesophageal reflux disease after fundoplicature in pediatric patients: a case-control study. *J. Pediatr. Surg.* 2007, 42, 1478-85.

[26] Kimber, C; Kiely, EM. The failure rate of surgery for gastroesophageal reflux. *J. Pediatr. Surg.* 1998, 33, 64-6.

[27] Esposito, C; Montupet, P. Long-term outcome of laparoscopic Nissen, Toupet, and Thal antireflux procedures for neurologically normal children with gastroesophageal reflux disease. *Surg. Endosc.* 2006, 20, 855-8.

[28] Capito, C; Leclair, MD. Long-term outcome of laparoscopic Nissen-Rossetti fundoplicature for neurologically impaired and normal children. *Surg. Endosc.* 2008, 22, 875-80.

[29] Pearl, RH; Robie, DK. Complications of gastroesophageal antireflux surgery in neurologically impaired versus neurologically normal children. *J. Pediatr. Surg.* 1990, 25, 1169-73.

[30] Lopez, M; Kalfa, N. Laparoscopic redo fundoplication in children. Failure causes and feasibility. *J. Pediatr. Surg.* 2008, 43, 1885-90.

[31] Fonkalsrud, EW; Bustorff-silva, J. Antireflux surgery in children under 3 months of age. *J. Pediatr. Surg.* 1999, 34, 527-31.

[32] Kubiak, R; Spitz, L. Effectiveness of fundoplicature in early infancy. *J. Pediatr. Surg.* 1999, 34, 295-99.

[33] Esposito, C; Montupet, P. Laparoscopic surgery for gastroesophageal reflux disease during the first year of life. *J. Pediatr. Surg.* 2001, 36, 715-17.

[34] Tovar, JA; Luis, AL. Pediatric surgeons and gastroesophageal reflux. *J. Pediatr. Surg.* 2007, 42, 277-83.

[35] Schols, AMWJ. Nutrition and outcome in chronic respiratory disease. *Nutrition*, 1997, 13, 161-3.

[36] Budweiser, S; Meyer, K. Nutritional depletion and its relationship to respiratory impairment in patients with chronic respiratory failure due to COPD or restrictive thoracic diseases. *Eur. J. Clin. Nutr.* 2008, 62, 436-43.
[37] Kamata, S; Usui, N. Long-term follow-up of patients with high-risk congenital diaphragmatic hernia. *J. Pediatr. Surg.* 2005, 40, 1833-8.
[38] Van Meurs, KP; Robbins, ST. Congenital diaphragmatic hernia: long-term outcome in neonates treated with extracorporeal membrane oxygenation. *J. Pediatr. Surg.* 1993, 122, 893-9.
[39] Jaillard, SM; Pierrat, V. Outcome at 2 years of infants with congenital diaphragmatic hernia: a population-based study. *Ann. Thorac. Surg.* 2003, 75, 250-6.
[40] Lund, DP; Mitchell, J. Congenital diaphragmatic hernia : the hidden morbidity. *J. Pediatr. Surg.* 1994, 29, 258-62.
[41] Cortes, RA; Keller, RL. Survival of severe congenital diaphragmatic hernia has morbid consequences. *J. Pediatr. Surg.* 2005, 40, 36-46.
[42] Cribbs, RK; Heiss, KF. Gastric fundoplicature is effective in promoting weight gain in children with severe congenital heart defects. *J. Pediatr. Surg.* 2008, 43, 283-9.
[43] Houtkooper, LB; Going, SB. Bioelectrical impedance estimation of fat-free body mass in children and youth: a cross-validation study. *J. Appl. Physiol.* 1992, 72, 366-73.
[44] Schaefer, F; Georgi, M. Usefulness of bioelectrical impedance and skinfold measurements in predicting fat-free mass derived from total body potassium in children. *Pediatr. Res.* 1994, 35, 617-24.
[45] Pichard, C; Kyle, UG. Fat-free mass in chronic illness: comparison of bioelectrical impedance and dual-energy X-ray absorptiometry in 480 chronically ill and healthy subjects. *Nutrition* 1999, 15, 668-76.
[46] Nakayama, DK; Motoyama, EK. Pulmonary function in newborns after repair of congenital diaphragmatic hernia. *Pediatr. Pulmonol.* 1991, 11, 49-55.
[47] Boas, SR; Kurland, G. Evolution of hyperresponsiveness in infants with severe congenital diaphragmatic hernia. *Pediatr. Pulmonol.* 1996, 22, 295-304.
[48] Harding, SM; Sontag, SJ. Asthma and gastroesophageal reflux. *Am. J. Gastroenterol.* 2000, 95, S23-32.
[49] Boesch, RP; Daines, C. Advances in the diagnosis and management of chronic pulmonary aspiration in children. *Eur. Respir. J.* 2006, 28, 847-61.

[50] Ahrens, P; Noll, C. Lipid-laden alveolar macrophages (LLAM): a useful marker of silent aspiration in children. *Pediatr. Pulmonol.* 1999, 28, 83-8.
[51] Harding, SM; Schan, CA. Gastroesophageal reflux-induced bronchoconstriction. Is microaspiration a factor? *Chest*, 1995, 108, 1220-7.
[52] Thilmany, C; Beck-Ripp, J. Acid and non-acid gastro-esophageal refluxes in children with chronic pulmonary diseases. *Respir. Med.* 2007, 101, 969-76.
[53] Vandenplas, Y; Salvatore, S. Gastro-esophageal reflux disease: impedance versus pH monitoring. *Acta Paediatr.* 2007, 96, 956-62.
[54] Field, SK; Sutherland, LR. Does medical anti-reflux therapy improve asthma in asthmatics with gastroesophageal reflux: a critical review of the litterature. *Chest,* 1998, 114, 275-83.
[55] Bowrey, DJ; Peters, JH. Gastroesophageal reflux disease in asthma. Effects of medical and surgical antireflux therapy on asthma control. *Ann. Surg.* 2000, 231, 161-72.
[56] Ahrens, P; Heller, K. Antireflux surgery in children suffering from reflux-associated respiratory diseases. *Pediatr. Pulmonol.* 1999, 28, 89-93.
[57] Tashjian, DB; Tirabassi, MV. Laparoscopic Nissen fundoplicature for reactive airway disease. *J. Pediatr. Surg.* 2002, 37, 1021-23.
[58] Mattioli, G; Bax, K. European multicenter survey on the laparoscopic treatment of gastroesophageal reflux in patients aged less than 12 months with supraesophageal symptoms. *Surg. Endosc.* 2005, 19, 1309-14.

Appendix

The following teams from the French CDH Study Group participating in this work: E. Carricaburu, MD, Department of Pediatric Surgery, Robert Debré Hospital, AP-HP, Paris; C. Chamond, MD, Department of Pediatric Surgery, Saint-Vincent de Paul Hospital, AP-HP, Paris; P. de Lagausie, MD, PhD, Department of Pediatric Surgery, University Hospital Timone Enfant, Marseille; M. Larroquet, MD, Department of Pediatric Surgery, Armand Trousseau Hospital, AP-HP, Paris; G. Levard, MD, PhD, Department of Pediatric Surgery, University Hospital la Miletrie, Poitiers; R. Sfeir, MD, Department of Pediatric Surgery, University Hospital Jeanne de Flandre, Lille; and D. Weil, MD, Department of Pediatric Surgery, Centre Hospitalier, Le Mans.

In: Hernias: Types, Symptoms and Treatment
Editor: James H. Wagner

ISBN: 978-1-61324-125-7
© 2011 Nova Science Publishers, Inc.

Chapter 5

Hiatal Hernias: Classification, Pathophysiology and Treatment

*Lourdes Robles, Christopher S. Davis
and P. Marco Fisichella**
Department of Surgery, Stritch School of Medicine,
Loyola University Medical Center, Maywood, Illinois, USA

Abstract

The purpose of this chapter is to comprehensively review hiatal hernias, with particular attention paid to their pathophysiology and available treatment strategies. In this chapter, the Authors will dedicate a section discussing the dominant theories regarding the pathogenesis of hiatal hernias at the molecular and cellular level.

In addition, the Authors will review the surgical treatment strategies and their indications, with a particular emphasis on the indications for surgery which have changed drastically in recent years. Overall, there are two basic types of hiatal hernias, sliding and paraesophageal, each with a wide array of symptoms ranging from benign or asymptomatic to severe and fatal.

---

*Department of Surgery, Stritch School of Medicine, Loyola University Medical Center, 2160 South First Avenue - Room 3226. Maywood, IL 60153, Phone: (708) 327-2236, Fax: (708) 327-3492

The most common symptoms observed are gastroesophageal reflux and dysphasia, and the treatment strategies employed are in large part to reduce the effects of these conditions while avoiding hernia recurrence.

Indeed, recent advancements in minimally invasive surgery have made the management of hiatal hernias radically different than a decade ago. Finally, the Authors will review the outcomes of surgical repairs including open, laparoscopic, and robotic approaches, and discuss the use of prosthetic meshes as an adjunct to the surgical treatment of this condition.

Introduction

The esophagus is a neuromuscular tube that functions as a conduit for the passage of food from the pharynx to the stomach. Approximately, 25-30 cm in length, the esophagus passes through the diaphragm at the level of the tenth thoracic vertebrae. The gastroesophageal (GE) junction prevents the reflux of gastric contents by a combination of methods including the approximation of the diaphragmatic crura, the baseline pressure of the lower esophageal sphincter, and the angle of His, which is formed by the gastric cardia and the distal esophagus. There are two main types of esophageal hernias: 1) the sliding hiatal hernia, and 2) the paraesophageal hernia. Hiatal hernias are relatively common and the majority do not cause any symptoms; in fact, the majority of hiatal hernias are found incidentally on imaging. In other patients, however, a hiatal hernia can be the cause of severe gastroesophageal reflux disease (GERD) along with its complications. Paraesophageal hernias, in contrast, have a normal GE junction and generally do not predispose a person to GERD, yet they carry a high risk of life threatening incarceration.

The treatment strategies can be divided into two main categories, medical management and surgical interventions. GERD management has vastly changed with the advent of proton pump inhibitors (PPIs), with an increase in patients being managed conservatively than in the past.

Not only has medical management of GERD improved in recent years but the surgical treatments available have drastically changed over the last decade with the popularization of laparoscopic surgery. Young patients or patients with complications associated with reflux disease can be treated successfully with surgery with improved outcomes, relatively low morbidity, and a lower risk of recurrence. The three major types of surgical approaches can be done open or through laparoscopy and include the Nissen fundoplication, Belsey (Mark IV), and the Hill repair. Ongoing advances have produced different strategies, as well as the implementation of different surgical aids to improve surgical outcomes and prevent recurrences.

Esophageal Hernia Types

Diaphragmatic hernias can be either congenital or acquired, with the latter being of traumatic or non-traumatic etiology. There are four types of acquired esophageal hernias. The Type I hiatal hernia, also known as a sliding hiatal hernia, comprises 95% of all hiatal herniations. This type of hernia occurs when a portion of the stomach prolapses through the diaphragmatic hiatus, thereby disrupting the normal location of the gastroesophageal junction. This disruption compromises the reflux barrier in terms of a reduced lower esophageal sphincter pressure, decreased pressure in the chest compared to the stomach, and also a reduction in acid clearance. Next, a type II hernia is known as a paraesophageal hernia or a rolling-type hernia. This hernia occurs when the fundus of the stomach prolapses into the chest through a widened diaphragmatic hiatus lateral to the esophagus. Though the GE junction remains intact, paraesophageal hernias have an increased risk of strangulation. Further, a Type III hernia is a combination of Types I and II with a sliding component and a paraesophageal hernia. Finally, a Type IV is a complex paraesophageal hernia where other abdominal contents along with the stomach are prolapsed into the chest cavity.

Pathogenesis of Hiatal Hernias

The pathogenesis of hiatal hernias continues to be poorly described and their true cause is likely multifactorial. As such, there appear to be three dominant theories underlying the pathogenesis of hiatal hernias: 1) increased intra-abdominal pressure that displaces the GE junction upward into the thorax; 2) esophageal shortening from congenital causes or acquired secondary to fibrosis; and 3) widening of the hiatus from congenital or acquired molecular and cellular changes in the crural muscles or connective tissue of the diaphragm.

Different studies have interrogated the correlation between obesity, the associated increased intra-abdominal pressure, and the rising incidence of hiatal hernias. [1,2,3,4] For instance, Sudhir et al found the endoscopic prevalence of a hiatal hernia was significantly higher in a morbidly obese group (BMI > 40 kg/m2) compared to a control group (BMI < 40 kg/m2). [4] Similarly, Pandolfino et al observed 285 obese patients and found that there was an increased intra-gastric and intra-esophageal pressure based on manometric studies compared to patients with a normal BMI. Their results showed an increase in anatomic separation between the LES and the crural diaphragm, which in turn predisposed these patients to developing hiatal hernias. [1]

In regards to esophageal shortening, a study from the 1970's in animal models showed a correlation between esophageal shortening caused by vagal stimulation and the formation of a hiatal hernia. [5] The pathogenesis behind the shortening includes prolonged fibrosis and scarring secondary to esophagitis. The newly shortened esophagus applies axial pressure on the GE junction promoting upward movement. Christensen et al studied the pathophysiology of this theory, concluding that reflux causes inflammation, edema, and fibrosis resulting in an inability to stretch the longitudinal muscles in the esophagus when a food bolus passes through the esophagus. [6]

Further evidence for the role of esophageal shortening and hiatal hernia formation is the positive outcomes in patients who undergo an elongation gastroplasty rather than a fundoplication procedure for repair of a hiatal hernia. [7, 8] The theory behind this form of repair is to eliminate the axial tension created, by elongating the esophagus.

The most objective evidence for the pathogenesis of hiatal hernia formation exists in support of changes at the cellular level to the connective tissues and muscles of the hernia complex. Hundreds of studies have been done to investigate the cellular and molecular causes of hernias. One study by Loukas et al examined 200 cadavers with hiatal hernias and observed the muscular contributions from the bilateral crura.

He found that most of the muscular contribution in the formation of the esophageal hiatus arose solely from the right crura. This is in contrast to a cadaver without herniation which revealed muscular contributions from both the right and left crura. They believed these variations could play a role hernia formation. [9] There is a strong correlation seen from various studies done in patients with inguinal and incisional hernias between the decreased ratio of type I "mature" collagen and type II "immature" collagen.

However, there are no studies as of yet that have looked at the collagen distribution in hiatal hernias, though it could be ascertained that a similar shift in collagen fibers exists. Evidence for this theory comes from a 2009 Swedish study whose authors discovered an abnormal collagen gene in 36 families that had a strong prevalence of GERD. These families were found to have an over expression of the gene COL3A1. COL3A1 is a gene on chromosome 2 that encodes for type II collagen, suggesting that abnormal collagen deposition strongly contributes to the formation of a hiatal hernia. [10]

Treatment

The treatment depends on the type of hernia, but in general, the approaches are either medical management or surgical intervention. Medical management includes lifestyle changes, dietary restrictions, and the use of acid suppressing drugs. Additionally, the majority of patients who were managed with surgery in the past are now successfully managed today with PPIs.

Gastroesophageal reflux is caused by the movement of gastric contents into the esophagus causing symptoms of reflux and injury to the esophageal mucosa. PPIs inhibit gastric acid secretion and increase the pH of the stomach. They do so by binding to the alpha subunit of the $H+/K+$ ATPase enzyme and irreversibly inhibiting acid production in about 70% of active pumps. [11] Sustained treatment with PPI's has been proven extremely efficacious for the prevention of GERD symptoms and minimizing esophageal mucosal injury. They are general well tolerated and have a low side effect profile, though for most patients a PPI is required for long-term use. Recent studies have investigated the implications of long-term use of PPIs and the possible complications. For example, studies have investigated a possible link between PPIs and infectious diseases such as pneumonia and pseudomembranous colitis, suggesting and increased prevalence in infection rate in patients taking acid suppressing drugs. [12, 13, 14] However, this correlation has not been substantiated in direct observational studies. [15, 16, 17] Another risk is the affect of PPIs on the body's ability to absorb calcium which can in turn lead to fractures. Along these lines, a study from the University of Manitoba showed the continuous use of PPIs for 5 years resulted in an increased risk of hip fractures. [17]

Overall, studies have determined that PPIs are effective and largely safe, but with the increasing popularity of minimally invasive surgery the debate has now turned to the cost effectiveness and quality of life differences between medical and surgical management. The multicenter REFLUX trial was a randomized study that compared laparoscopic surgery with continued medical management for patients with GERD. At one year follow-up, a significant increase in quality of life was observed in the surgical group compared to the medicine group. Quality of life was based on a 36 item questionnaire developed specifically for the study. [18] An example of the long-term success of laparoscopic hiatal hernia repair was recently reported by Furnee et al, who found that 89% of patients rated their symptoms as resolved or improved after surgery, while only 12% experienced post-operative daily heart burn and/or dysphagia.[19] Finally, Cookson et al concluded that laparoscopic surgery had similar costs compared to medical management at eight years with cost-savings thereafter.[20] These results were recently supported by a similar study that found surgery to be cost effective assuming effects lasted for at least five years and patients who failed surgery did not have worse symptoms than before surgical intervention. [21] There is good evidence to support the increased quality of life and cost effectiveness of surgical intervention but because of their efficacy and safety profile the American Gastroenterological Association continues to recommend an initial trial of PPI with surgery offered as an alternative. [22] As such, what may be most appropriate would be to tailor therapy based on the age of the patient, the presence of changes in the esophageal mucosa, and the need for long term medicine use to decide if surgery is the more appropriate initial treatment.

Surgical Treatments

Laparoscopic surgery represents the gold standard in surgical management of GERD and dysphagia with or without the presence of a hernia. For symptomatic hiatal hernias virtually all surgical interventions involve repair of the diaphragmatic hiatus and a gastric wrap around the esophagus. The three most common approaches for surgical repair of hiatal hernias are the Nissen, the Belsey (Mark IV), and the Hill repairs. The Nissen fundoplication involves repair of the diaphragmatic hiatus and a 360 degree fundic wrap around the GE junction. The Belsey (Mark IV) fundoplication involves a 270 wrap and approximation of the left and right crura of the diaphragm. The Hill repair anchors the gastric cardia to the posterior abdomen, which in effect augments the angle of his. The initial steps for any hiatal hernia repair are essentially the same. The hiatal hernia is reduced and the hernia sac is dissected off of the crura. The fundus of the stomach is mobilized from the spleen and diaphragm and the short gastrics are divided. Once the gastric fundus is well mobilized it can be used to form the wrap around the esophagus.

Today, the Nissen fundoplication is considered the primary surgical intervention for the treatment of symptomatic hiatal hernias. The procedure was first performed by Dr. Rudolph Nissen in 1955, gained popularity in the 1970s, and was adopted laparoscopically in the early 1990s. One study reported that after 10 years, 89.5% of patients were still symptom-free.[23] The technique involves mobilization of the esophagus through a transhiatal incision, division of the short gastric vessels to mobilize the gastric fundus, and a tension free 360 degree fundoplication that essentially recreates a high pressure zone and prevents reflux of gastric contents into the esophagus. The complications associated with this surgery include dysphasia, "gas bloating syndrome," and recurrence or wrap migration. [24] Over time the Nissen fundoplication has undergone many alterations aimed at improving some of the complications and side-effects of the original surgical repair. For instance, critics of this procedure cite an increased incidence of dysphagia in patients undergoing a full wrap; however, this has largely been improved with the use of a larger boogie placed into the esophagus to tighten the wrap. Nonetheless, controversy persists as to the best operative technique, specifically as it relates to full (Nissen) vs partial (Toupet) fundoplication. Compared to a Nissen fundoplication, a Toupet repair involves anchoring the posterior wall of the fundus behind the esophagus to the right side causing a posterior partial wrap around the esophagus. Recently, Wenk et al showed equal rates of reflux control but a lower complication rate with the Toupet fundoplication. [25] Based on these results and those of others some centers exclusively do partial fundoplications while other centers tailor their treatments based on patient's symptoms.

Another widely debated topic is the use of mesh to re-enforce a hiatal hernia repair. One study by Sorcelli retrospectively compared three different methods for performing a fundoplication in 297 patients treated from 1992 to 2007. One group of patients received crural closure using suture alone, the second group received closure using a polyprolene mesh, and the last group received suture closure plus a superimposed tailored mesh. The results revealed a 9.6% post-operative hernia recurrence or wrap migration in patients that underwent suture only hiatoplasty, compared to only 1.8% in patients that received mesh only. There was no statically significant difference between patients that received mesh only repair and suture with superimposed mesh repair. [26] The concern for the use of mesh during surgical repair is the possibility for erosion and a highly morbid perforation. Yet, in the study of Sorcelli et al, a mesh-related complication occurred in only one patient (0.49%). This patient suffered a gastric perforation which was managed intraoperatively with no further complications. [26] The low morbidity rate has also been observed in other similar studies. [27, 28, 29, 30] This lead the authors to conclude that prosthetic related complications during a very long follow-up is very low and therefore the use of mesh is a safe and effective means to provide satisfactory outcomes. [26, 30]

Another well known complication associated with any fundoplication surgery is hernia recurrence. In the past it was believed that when a primary laparoscopic hitalplasty failed the treatment strategy involved an open revision. During the 1990s, however, more surgeons began performing laparoscopic revision fundoplications. Most patients that underwent these revisions required complete reconstruction of the fundoplication with removal and placement of new sutures. Excellent outcomes were observed with laparoscopic repairs, making it the procedure technique of choice for recurrent hernias. [31]

Similar to the vast changes in hiatal hernia repairs in the last decade, the repair of paraesophageal hernias have also evolved over time. Until recently the treatment of both symptomatic and asymptomatic paraesophageal hernias involved urgent surgical repair to prevent the life-threatening complications of obstruction and strangulation. This has been called into question by several studies, and the routine repair of paraesophageal hernias is no longer supported. Now a more conservative philosophy has been adopted, promoting a watchful waiting approach. [30, 32]

Other treatment evolutions for paraesophageal hernias involve the use of mesh to reinforce the repair. In one prospective randomized trial comparing simple cruroplasty versus mesh there was a 22 % recurrence rate with suture repair compared to 0 % in the mesh group. [30] Additionally, though the rate of complications with the use of mesh is small, when they do occur they can be life-threatening and involve the morbidity of total gastrectomy or esophagectomy. For these grave complications the use of biological prosthesis has gained popularity. The difficulty, however, is that there is no well described method for securing a biologic mesh. To address this concern, Tayyab et al used a piece of porcine intestinal submucosa as a mesh for their hernia repairs. Their method of securing the mesh involved suturing through the mesh and then to the base of the left crus followed by the base of the right crus and then into the mesh. This was repeated until the crura were closed to the posterior margin of the esophagus, usually requiring three horizontal mattress stitches. With this technique the mesh would lay flat across the crura. In their study of over 150 cases, only one patient had a recurrence. Finally, though there were three intraoperative complications and seven postoperative complications, none were associated with the use of mesh. [33]

While most centers are employing mesh into their paraesophageal hernia repairs, its use continues to be debated among some surgeons. The belief is that herniation is associated with two different processes: 1) tension caused by the migration of the GE junction in the setting of an acquired short esophagus; and 2) tension outward on the hiatus as the hernia enlarges. The goal of mesh repair is to oppose the radial tension by strengthening the hiatal orifice. Some surgeons however, believe that axial tension can be eliminated by an esophageal lengthening procedure. The initial dissection technique of a Collis gastroplasty is essentially identical to that used for an uncomplicated fundoplication. After mobilization of the gastric fundus a Penrose drain encircles the esophagus. Dissection continues into the mediastinum for 4–6 cm. A full thickness incision of the gastric cardia is created with a staple line paralleled to the lesser curvature with occasional reinforcement of the staple line with vertical mattress sutures. This technique serves to lengthen the esophagus by creating a tube out of the upper portion of the stomach.[7] A recently published retrospective study had the largest series to date of esophageal lengthening procedures. 63% of patient underwent an esophageal lengthening procedure with good outcomes in up to 90% of patients. The authors did note, however, that the trend over the recent years was towards the use of mesh and that patient's comorbid factors were found to be worse presently compared to the past, leaving the use of mesh as a topic for further research. [34]

Evolving Treatments

A case report by DeUgarte et al in 2009 illustrated the repair of a congenital paresophageal hiatal hernia on a 3 year old child utilizing a da Vinci robot. The patient had complete resolution of her symptoms; however, the cost of the operation was significantly increased and the operation had a prolonged setup and procedural time with a surgeon required at the bedside to aid in retraction. Nonetheless, their opinion regarding the use of robotics in esophageal hernias was favorable and with continued streamlining of robotics in surgical intervention the utilization of resources should improve. [35]

References

[1] Pandolfino JE, EL-Serag HB, Shah N, Ghosh SK, Kahrillas PJ. Obestity: a challenge to esophagogastric junction integrity. *Gastroenterology* 2006; 130: 988-999.
[2] Fass R. The pathophysiologic mechanism of GERD in the obese patient. *Digestive Diseases and Sciences,* 2008; 53: 2300-2306.
[3] Sakaguchi MO, Hashimoto T, Asakuma Y, Takao M, Tsuji Y, Yamamoto N, Shimada M, Lee K, Ashida K. Obesity as a risk factor for GERD in Japan. *Journal of Gastroenterology,* 2008; 43: 57-62.
[4] Sadhir KD, Manish A, Agrawal K, Hany B, Alejandro G. Upper Gastrointestinal Symptoms and associated disorders in morbidly obese patients: A prospective study. *Digestive Diseases and Sciences,* 2009; 54: 1243-1246.
[5] Christensen J, Roustem M. Hiatus Hernia: A review of evidence for its origin in esophageal longitudinal muscle dysfunction. *American Journal of Medicine,* 2000; 108: 3-7.
[6] Dodds WJ, Stewart ET, Hedges D, Zboralske FF. Movement of the feline esophagus associated with respiration and peristalsis. *Journal of Clinical Investigation,* 1973; 52: 1-13.
[7] Johnson AB, Oddsdottir M, Hunter JG. Laparoscopic Collis gastroplasty and Nissen fundiplication. *Surgical Endoscopy,* 1998; 12- 1055-1060.
[8] D'Journo, XB, Martin J, Bensaidane, S, Ferraro P, Duranceau A. Elongation gastroplasty with transverse fundoplasty: The Jeyasingham repair. *Journal of Thoracic and Cardiovascular Surgery,* 2009; 138: 1192-1199.
[9] Loukas MW, Tubbs RS, Louis RG, Gupta AA, Jordan R. Morphologic variation of the diaphragmatic crura: a correlation with pathologic processes of the esophageal hiatus? *Folia Morphologica,* 2008; 67: 273-279.
[10] Asling B, Jirholt J, Hammond P, Knutsson M, Walentinsson A, Davisdon G. Collagen type III alpha I is a gastro-oesophageal reflux susceptibility gene and a male risk factor for hiatus hernia. *Gut,* 2009; 58: 1063-1069.
[11] Katz OP, Zavala S. Proton Pump Inhibitors in the management of GERD. *J. of Gastrointestinal Surg.* 2009; 14: 62-66.
[12] Howell MD, Novack V, Grgurich P, Soulliard D, Novack L, Pencina M, Talmor D. Iatrogenic gastric acid suppression and the risk of nosocomial

Clostridium difficile infection. *Archives of Internal Medicine* 2010; 170: 784-790.
[13] Restrepo MI, Mortensen EM, Anzueto A. Common medications that increase the risk for developing community-acquired pneumonia. *Current Opinion in Infectious Disease*, 2010; 23: 145-151.
[14] Eurich DT, Sadowski CA, Simpson SH, Marrie TJ, Majumdar SR. Recurrent community-acquired pneumonia in patients starting acid-suppressing drugs. *The American Journal of Medicine*, 2010; 123: 47-53.
[15] Beaulieu M, Williamson D, Sirois C, Lachaine J. Do proton-pump inhibitors increase the risk for nosocomial pneumonia in a medical intensive care unit? *Journal of Critical Care*, 2008; 23: 513-518.
[16] Sultan N, Nazareno J, Gregor J. Association between proton pump inhibitors and respiratory infections: a systematic review and meta-analysis of clinical trials. *Canadian Journal of Gastroenterology,* 2008; 22: 761-766.
[17] Harvard Health Fellows. Do PPIs have Long Term Side Effects? Harvard Health Publication 2009; 4-6.
[18] Wileman GA, Ramsay C, Bojke L, Espstein D, Schulpher M, Macran S, Kilonzo M, Vale L, Francis J, Mowat A, Krukowski Z, Heading R, Thursz M, Russell I. Campbell M. The effectiveness and cost-effectiveness of minimal access surgery amongst people with gastro-oesophageal reflux disease- a UK collaborative study. The REFLUX trial. *Helath Technology Assessment*, 2008; 12: 1-181.
[19] Furnee E, Draaisma W, Simmermacher R, Stapper G, Broeders I. Long-term symptomatic outcome and radiologic assessment of laparoscopic hiatal hernia repair. *American Journal of Surgery*, 2010; 199: 695-701.
[20] Cookson R, Flood C, Koo B, Mahon D, Rhodes M. Short term cost effectiveness and long term cost analysis comparing laparoscopic Nissen fundoplication with proton-pump inhibitor maintenance for gastro-oesophageal reflux disease. *BJ Surg*. 2005; 92: 700-706.
[21] Epstein, D, Bojke L, Scupher M. Laparoscopic fundoplication compared with medical management for gastro-oesophageal reflux disease: cost effectiveness study. *BMJ*, 2009; 338: 1-7.
[22] Wileman SM, McCann S, Grant AM, Krukowski ZH, Bruce J. Medical versus surgical management for gastro-esophageal reflux disease in adults. *Cochrane Database Syst. Rev*. 2010; 3: 244-245.
[23] Minjarez R, Jobe B. Surgical therapy for gastroesophageal reflux disease. *GI Motility,* 2006; 1038: 1-35.

[24] DeMeester TR, Bonavina L, Albertucci M. Nissen fundoplication for gastroesophageal reflux disease. Evaluation of primary repair in 100 consecutive patients. *Annals of Surgery*, 1986; 204: 9-20.
[25] Wenk C, Zornig C. Laparoscopic Toupet fundiplication. *Langenbecks Arch. Surgery*, 2010; 395; 459-461.
[26] Soricelli E, Basso N, Genco A, Cipriano M. Long-term results of hiatal hernia mesh repair and antirelux laparoscopic surgery. *Surgical Endoscopy*, 2009; 23: 2499-2504.
[27] Carlson MA, Franizides CT. Complications and results of primary minimally invasive antireflux procedures: a review of 10,735 reported cases. *Journal of American College of Surgeons*, 2001; 193: 428-437.
[28] Frantizides CT, Madan AT, Carlson MA, Stavropulous GP. A prospective randomized trial of laparoscopic polytetrafluoroethylene (PTFE) patch repair vs simple cruroplasty for large hiatal hernia. *Archives of Surgery*, 2002; 137: 649-652.
[29] Stadlhuber RJ, Sherif AE, Mittal SK et al. Mesh complications after prosthetic reinforcement of hiatal closure: a 28 case series. *Journal of Surgical Endoscopy*, 2008; 10: 205-207.
[30] Patti M, Fisichella P. Laparascopic Paraesophageal hernia repair. How I do it. *J. gastrointestinal surgery* 2009; 13: 1728-1732.
[31] Frantzides C, Madan A, Carlson M, Zeni T, Zografakis J, Moore R, Meiselman M, Luu M, Ayiomamitis G. *Laparascopic revision of failed fundiplication and hital herniorrhaphy.*
[32] Larusson HJ, Zingg U, Hahnloser D, Delport K, Seifert B, Oertli D. Predictive factors for morbidity and mortality in patients undergoing laparoscopic Paraesophageal hernia repair: Age, ASA score and operation type influence morbidity. *World J. Surgery*, 2009; 33: 980-985.
[33] Diwan T, Martinec D, Ujiki M, Dunst C, Swanstrom L. A simplified technique for placement of biologic mesh in paraesophageal hernia repair. *Surgical Endoscopy*, 2010; 24: 221-222.
[34] Luketich et al. Outcomes after a decade of laparoscopic giant paraesophageal hernia repair. *Journal of Thoracic and cardiovascular surgery* 2010; 139: 395-405.
[35] DeUgarte D, Hirschl R, Geiger J. Robotic repair of congenital paraesophageal hiatal hernia: Case Report. *J. of Laparoendoscopic and advanced surgical techniques* 2009; 19: 187-189.

In: Hernias: Types, Symptoms and Treatment ISBN: 978-1-61324-125-7
Editor: James H. Wagner © 2011 Nova Science Publishers, Inc.

Chapter 6

The Applicability, Alternation and Future Research in Laparoscopic Surgery for Pediatric Inguinal Hernias

Yu-Tang Chang[*]

Division of Pediatric Surgery, Department of Surgery,
Kaohsiung Medical University Hospital, Kaohsiung Medical University,
100 Tzyou 1st Road, Kaohsiung, 80708 Taiwan

Abstract

Laparoscopic surgery for pediatric inguinal hernia has been performed for over one-and-a-half decades. Numerous laparoscopic approaches have been reported, including intracorporeal ligation of the hernia defect with or without separation of the distal sac, and percutaneous endoscopically assisted ligation of the defect by variable devices.

However, there is no single laparoscopic approach that has fully replaced conventional inguinal herniotomy, since recurrence rate after laparoscopic surgery is generally known to be higher than after conventional inguinal herniotomy.

---

[*]Tel. 886-7-3121101-6303, Fax: 886-7-3127056, E-mail: 890300@ms.kmuh.org.tw

This chapter comprehensively reviews and compares the various laparoscopic techniques. There is a tendency toward diminishing the size and number of abdominal incisions and decreasing the usage of endoscopic instrumentation.

Single-port endoscopic-assisted percutaneous extraperitoneal closure seems to be the ultimate attainment. Technical evolution involving complete enclosure of the hernia defect without peritoneal gaps, the utility of preperitoneal hydrodissection, ligation of the defect with division of the distal sac, and double-ligation of the defect seems to be sufficient to achieve a low recurrence rate.

The future development of the technique is to move towards little invasiveness without complications, easy manipulation for widespread adoption, and recognition as a gold standard for the treatment of pediatric inguinal hernia.

Introduction

Inguinal hernia in infancy and childhood is one of the most common surgical conditions managed by pediatric surgeons [1,2]. Pediatric inguinal hernia is almost exclusively an indirect type because it is formed by failure of obliteration of the processus vaginalis in the male and the canal of Nuck in the female.

The processus vaginalis is present during the third month of gestation. It accompanies the gubernaculum and the testis during their descent through the inguinal canal and reaches the scrotum by the seventh month of intrauterine life.

In the female, the canal extends along the round ligament. Obliteration of the processus vaginalis usually commences soon after the descent of the testis is completed and continues after birth.

However, incomplete obliteration of the processus vaginalis may predispose various patterns of fluid accumulation (hydrocele) and hernia (Figure 1). Since an inguinal hernia does not resolve spontaneously, surgical repair should be performed shortly after diagnosis on an elective basis. Inguinal herniotomy is a well-developed surgical technique for uncomplicated inguinal hernia in infants and children. The technique usually necessitates a small 1.5 to 2 cm inguinal incision and involves the separation of the hernia sac from the spermatic cord, high suture ligation of the separated sac doubly tied, and possible removal of the distal sac/hydrocele [1,2,3]. In most patients, the technique can be safely done in the outpatient surgical unit. The possible postoperative complications, such as recurrence or injury to the vas deferens in male children, are not high, and the scar is usually hidden in the skin crease [1].

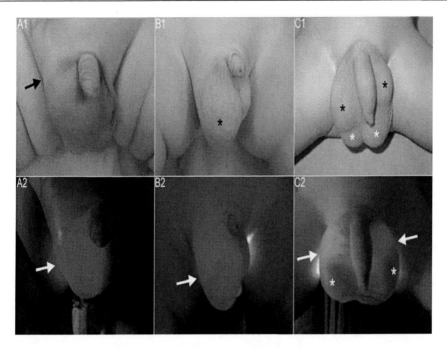

Figure 1. Different forms of inguinal hernia and hydrocele arising from failure of the processus vaginalis to obliterate completely. Note a right inguinal hernia with bowel incarceration (black arrow) in a 2-month-old male [A1], a right scrotal hydrocele (black asterisk) in a one-year-old male [B1], and bilateral hydroceles of the spermatic cord (black asterisks) located above the testis (white asterisks) in a 4-month-old male patient [C1]. With a flashlight placed behind these scrotal masses, all showed a positive transillumination (whites arrows) [A2, B2, C2], and transillumination of a scrotal mass may imply air, fluid or incarcerated bowel.

The Applicability of Laparoscopy to Pediatric Inguinal Hernia

During the last one-and-a-half decades, the conventional method of inguinal hernia repair has been challenged by technical refinements in the laparoscopic surgery [4,5,6]. The initial use of laparoscopy in the pediatric hernia patient was to examine the contralateral groin, either through a remotely placed port or the opened processus vaginalis, during open, unilateral hernia surgery [2,4]. In 1997, El-Gohary first described laparoscopic ligation of inguinal hernia in girls [7].

Moreover, the patency of the contralateral processus vvaginalis can be visualized and repaired simultaneously (Figure 2). Besides, laparoscopy can serve as a diagnostic and therapeutic tool in patients with a reducible cord hudrocele or a communicating hydrocele (Figure 3) [8,9].

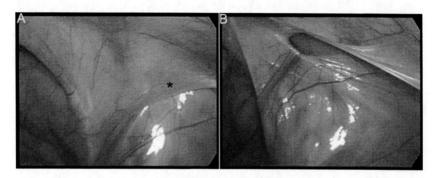

Figure 2. Note a 5-year-old female patient with a patent canal of Nuck during contralateral laparoscopic hernia repair. The orifice was obscured by a peritoneal fold (asterisk) [A] and was visualized after elevation of the peritoneal fold by an endoscopic forceps [B].

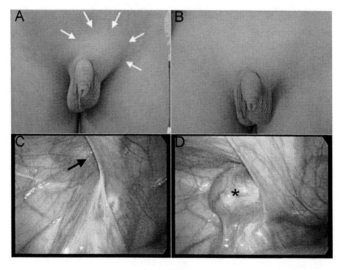

Figure 3. Note a reducible hydrocele of the spermatic cord in a 9-year-old boy. [A] In a standing position, left groin bulging (white arrows) is apparent. [B] Note spontaneous disappearance of the bulging in a lying position. Through laparoscopy, [C] a patent processus vaginalis (black arrow) was noted and [D] a hydrocele with integrated wall (asterisk) can be seen by external manual squeezing.

Subsequently, numerous technical reports for the laparoscopic hernia repair in children have been evolved [4]. These techniques vary considerably in their approaches to the hernia defect with/without division of the distal sac, use of ports (three, two, or one), assistant instrumentation (two, one, or none), suture materials (absorbable, nonabsorbable), closure of the defect (intraperitoneal, extra-peritoneal) and techniques of knot-tying (intracorporeal, extracorporeal) [4].

Compared to the conventional inguinal herniotomy, many authors have emphasized the advantage of laparoscopic repairs, including avoidance of injury to the vas deferens and testicular vessels, the absent manipulation of the cord structure, and the more correct diagnosis regarding associate direct and femoral hernias [4].

Technical Limitations of Laparoscopic Surgery for Pediatric Inguinal Hernia

Although the advantages of laparoscopic surgery have been well addressed, there is no single laparoscopic approach that has fully replaced conventional inguinal herniotomy. There are some technical limitations that influence a pediatric surgeon's willingness to perform the procedure. The known limitations of the laparoscopic surgery for pediatric inguinal hernia are as follows:

(1) *Laparoscopic surgery for pediatric inguinal hernia is generally thought not to be a minimally invasive surgery.* Conventional inguinal herniotomy is easily and efficaciously addressed. However, the laparoscopic approach, transforming a routine extraperitoneal procedure into a transperitoneal one may be considered contentious, as it may seem to make an easy surgery unnecessarily difficult because of the need of multiple abdominal incisions and pneumoperitoneum in the operating room. A true laparoscopic herniotomy may employ a laparoscope inserted via an umbilical incision and two lateral ports for instrumentation to dissect the hernia sac and ligate the defect [10,11,12,13]. The necessity for intraabdominal laparoscopic skills, such as intracorporeal suturing, knot-tying and manipulation of the suture on a needle may be time-consuming and cumbersome [13]. In a single-blinded, randomized study, recovery and outcome were similar after conventional inguinal herniotomy and laparoscopic herniotomy in children [14]. Compared to conventional inguinal herniotomy with an

almost disappeared wound in the skin crease, laparoscopic herniotomy did not achieve any superiority in cosmesis. Moreover, laparoscopic herniotomy was associated with increased operative time and postoperative pain [13,14].

(2) *Recurrence rate after laparoscopic surgery is generally known to be higher than after conventional inguinal herniotomy* [1,15]. Partial omission of the defect circumference, strength and appropriateness of the knot, inclusion of tissue other than peritoneum in the suture with a propensity for subsequent loosening, use of absorbable sutures, and failure to detect a rare or direct hernia are some reported factors contributing to recurrence in laparoscopic surgery [4]. However, most of these emerging techniques merely use a single suture to obliterate the defect extracorporeally or intracorporeally with neither separation of the hernia sac from the spermatic cord nor division with the distal sac, which go against every step of conventional inguinal herniotomy [4]. Moreover, since the vas deferens and testicular vessels are adherent to the hernia sac, these vital structures may be injured by their inclusion in the suture or may be left untouched (jump over them) during closure of the hernia defect (Figure 4) [4], possibly resulting in peritoneal gaps and has been reported as an important factor contributing to recurrence and postoperative hydrocele [4].

The Alternations of Laparoscopy in Pediatric Inguinal Hernia

The Alternation to Become a True Minimally Invasive Surgery

Modifications on the laparoscopic surgery for pediatric inguinal hernia continue to be refined, with a trend toward extracorporeal knot-tying and reduced incision size and number of ports [4]. Single-port laparoscopic-assisted percutaneous extraperitoneal closure, including subcutaneous endoscopically-assisted ligation (SEAL), and percutaneous internal ring suturing (PIRS), seems to be the ultimate attainment [6,16,17,18,19,20,21]. Under laparoscopic guide, the suture is introduced and withdrawn percutaneously at the level of the orifice of the hernia defect by variable devices, and is tied extracorporeally to obliterate the hernia sac. The knot is then placed in the subcutaneous space. Since these procedures were extracorporeal closure of the hernia sac, it also eliminated the need for intraabdominal laparoscopic skills. Only one umbilical trocar wound and groin needle puncture wounds were made (Figure 5). Therefore, the technique could provide better cosmetics and reach the state of minimally invasive surgery [22].

For lack of assistance of working instruments in the single-port laparoscopic technique, some authors may be concerned about the difficulty of removal of the soft suture thread out of the body [23]. Therefore, single umbilical incision laparoscopic-assisted percutaneous extraperitoneal closure is another option. Some surgeons perform a very similar hernia repair with an ureteroscope or addition of introducing an extra grasping instrument through the umbilicus alongside the telescope to assist with the purse-string suture [23,24].

However, with or without assistance of working instruments, there are some drawbacks in the single umbilical incision laparoscopic surgery for pediatric inguinal hernia. First, reported single-incision laparoscopic techniques are not laparoscopic herniotomy since the distal sac has never been divided. Recurrence rate/postoperative hydrocele may be high if the continuity of the peritoneum fails to be disrupted completely. Second, being a technique of percutaneous closure of inguinal hernia, simultaneous ligation of subcutaneous tissues between the skin and hernia sac may be inevitable [11,20]. Some authors may worry that inclusion of superfluous tissues in the ligature might possibly increase a propensity for subsequent loosening and later recurrence [4].

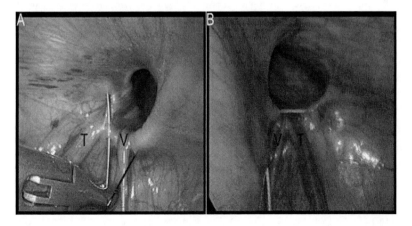

Figure 4. Peritoneal gaps occurred during laparoscopic hernia repair using the technique of either intraperitoneal suturing [A] or percutaneous extraperitoneal ligation [B]. Without the

assistance of preperitoneal hydrodissection, the needle and suture should bypass the vas deferens (V) and testicular vessels (T) to avoid injury to these vital structures.

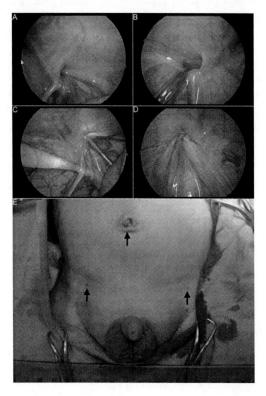

Figure 5. Intraoperative photo showing a 3-month-old male receiving one-trocar laparoscopic transperitoneal repair. [A,B] Right side inguinal hernia and contralateral patent processus vaginalis were noted. [C,D] Both defects were repaired simultaneously. [E] Postoperative picture showing the final wound appearance. According to the ruler placed below, the wounds (arrows) were minimal.

The Alternation to Reduce the Recurrence Rate

The inguinal hernia or patent processus vaginalis is an otupouching of the peritoneum through the inguinal canal [2]. From laparoscopic viewing of a treated inguinal hernia in children, local intraperitoneal adhesions at the original entrance of the hernia can be visualized after either conventional inguinal herniotomy or laparoscopic surgery (Figure 6) [6,15,25]. Since postsurgical peritoneal adhesions are a consequence of injured peritoneal surface (including incision, cauterization, suturing or other means of trauma) fusing together to form scar tissue [26], such adhesions after inguinal hernia repair may occur because of the healing process after dissection of the cord, suture ligation of the sac, and subsequent tissue reaction of the suture. Since the tensile strength of any suture material may diminish eventually, several authors suggested that peritoneal healing or reperitonealization may be the leading factor for complete obliteration of the hernia defect in the long run [6,25].

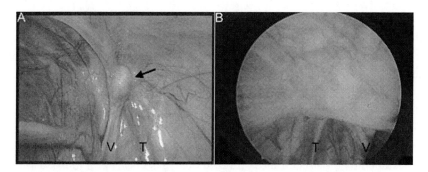

Figure 6. Laparoscopic views of inguinal hernia treated after conventional inguinal herniotomy [A] and laparoscopic surgery [B]. [A] Note local intraperitoneal adhesion and a stitch granuloma (arrow) at the original entrance into the hernia sac 13 months after conventional inguinal herniotomy in a 2-year-old male. [B] Laparoscopic surgery for other reasons was performed 56 days after laparoscopic left side herniorrhaphy in a 5-month-old male. Note the peritoneal scarring occurred in closure of the hernia defect.

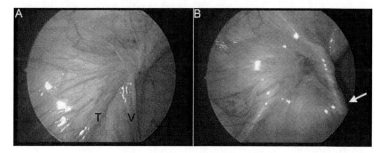

Figure 7. Intraoperative photo showing the "preperitoneal hydrodissection" method in a 3-year-old boy. [A] Note left side inguinal hernia and the close proximity of the vas deferens (V) and testicular vessels (T) to the ring. [B] Introduction of the vascular catheter (arrow) percutaneously into the preperitoneal space along right side of the hernia defect. Injection of normal saline via the vascular catheter helps to separate the vas and vessels from the peritoneum and enclose the defect without peritoneal gaps.

In the era of minimally invasive surgery, it is necessary to apply adequate peritoneal healing to any aspect of the hernia defect. It seems that even leaving a small peritoneal gap suffices to induce subsequent widening and hernia recurrence [4]. Therefore, completely enclosing the hernia defect without peritoneal gaps, the same as suture ligation in the conventional inguinal herniotomy, is crucial to reach a near-zero recurrence rate [6].

In 2004, Chan et al emphasized the importance of using a "complete ring sign", a complete ring of peritoneum without a visible significant portion of raw stitch, for prevent recurrence [5]. In addition, the method of preperitoneal hydrodissection, injection of normal saline in the extraperitoneal space at the level of internal inguinal ring (Figure 7), is helpful to separate the vas and vessels from the peritoneum; therefore, a completely enclosing suture for the hernia defect could be provided without jumping over or including these vital structures [5,20]. Since the preperitoneal space is filled with avascular fat tissue and loose areolar tissue, hydrodissection can be made very easily with a metal cannula or a vascular catheter [5,16,20,21,27]. In 2007, Chan and colleagues employed preperitoneal hydrodissection in the three-port intraperitoneal-suturing technique, and concluded that the recurrence rate could decrease from 4.88 to 0.4% after the usage of preperitoneal hydrodissection [27]. Recently, the method of preperitoneal hydrodissection has been applied in the single-port technique [16,20,21]. Meanwhile, the method of preperitoneal hydrodissection is useful in (i) providing additional space for negotiating the working instruments; (ii) keeping the device just under the peritoneum, and observing the needle sign [5,27]; (iii) avoiding injury to the vas and vessels; (iv) separating the sac from the spermatic cord; (v) enabling further tensionless knot-tying [27] ; and (vi) decreasing postoperative hydrocele [16], which may be caused by interruption of testicular lymphatic drainage because of being thicker than the peritoneum bites of the encircling suture [6]. Moreover, normal saline, the solution for preperitoneal hydrodissection, could predispose the formation of peritoneal adhesions and fibrosis [28]. Therefore, during passing of the suture, preperitoneal normal saline injection may cause more tissue trauma, further promoting the formation of peritoneal adhesions and minimizing later recurrence.

In order to lower the recurrence rate, some authors follow every step of conventional inguinal herniotomy in the laparoscopic surgery: dissection, division and suture ligation of the processus vaginalis at the internal ring [10,11,12,13]. However, in either the three-port laparoscopic herniotomy with intracorporeal knot-tying or two-port technique with an assistant port for intraabdominal suturing [15,29], the hernia defect is always closed by N-shaped or purse-string sutures, both of which cannot enclose the defect completely and may leave multiple peritoneal gaps [30]. Reported recurrences have usually occurred in close proximity to the vas as well as the testicular and inferior epigastric vessels medially to the previous suture [30]. Therefore, division of the hernia sac at the level of the internal ring is the most important step to avoid recurrence when laparoscopic herniotomy is adopted [25]. In 2010, Riquelme and colleagues also demonstrated that it is not necessary to ligate the hernia defect after division of the sac if the width of hernia defect is small than 10mm [25].

If suture ligation is the only method without any division of the sac, the author suggests that it is necessary to provide a complete extraperitoneal enclosing suture for the defect. With the aid of preperitoneal hydrodissection, single-port laparoscopic percutaneous extraperitoneal closure may be the preferred technique. Moreover, in the single-port technique, the ligation of the hernia defect could be achieved percutaneously without the need for intraabdominal manipulation of the needle and intracorporeal knot-tying [20].

However, laparoscopic techniques for pediatric inguinal hernia almost always rely on one suture to obliterate the hernia defect [4]. A single enclosing suture may be enough if tensile strength of the knot could be maintained until peritoneal healing. However, a second or even third suture may be applied if the hernia defect was considered to be incompletely closed by the first suture [16]. Although the fear of impairing testicular perfusion is unfounded [31], it has been shown that a scheme for complete enclosure of the hernia defect should be planned before operation. In 2010, Lipskar et al first described laparoscopic double-ligation of inguinal hernia in girls [32]. However, in male children, the technique of laparoscopic double-ligation as a routine procedure has never been reported.

Future Prospects

To enhance pediatric surgeons' willingness to perform the procedure, a simple and safe laparoscopic technique should be designed. The necessity of performing a true laparoscopic herniotomy or other complicated intraperitoneal techniques may be reconsidered. Ideal laparoscopic inguinal hernia repair should be minimally invasiveness without complications, easily manipulable for widespread adoption, and ineluctably moving toward a gold standard for the treatment of pediatric inguinal hernia.

Completely extraperitoneal enclosing the hernia defect with preperitoneal hydrodissection could decrease peritoneal gaps, and single-port endoscopic-assisted percutaneous extraperitoneal closure may be the preferred technique. The method of preperitoneal hydrodissection could help to completely enclose the hernia defect without peritoneal gaps. Furthermore, the smaller and fewer skin incisions of the single-port laparoscopic surgery could reach the state of minimally invasive surgery. However, single-port laparoscopic surgery for pediatric inguinal hernia is a technique in evolution. More long-term follow-up concerning the recurrence rate is necessary.

References

[1] Ein SH, Njere I, Ein A. Six thousand three hundred sixty-one pediatric inguinal hernias: a 35-year review. *J. Pediatr. Surg.* 2006;41:980-986.
[2] International Pediatric Endosurgery Group. IPEG Guidelines for Inguinal Hernia and Hydrocele. *J. Laparoendosc. Adv. Surg. Tech. A.* 2010;20:x-xiv.
[3] Mohta A, Jain N, Irniraya KP, Saluja SS, Sharma S, Gupta A. Non-ligation of the hernial sac during herniotomy: a prospective study. *Pediatr. Surg. Int.* 2003;19:451-452.
[4] Saranga Bharathi R, Arora M, Baskaran V. Minimal access surgery of pediatric inguinal hernias: a review. *Surg. Endosc.* 2008;22:1751-1762.
[5] Chan KL, Tam PK. Technical refinements in laparoscopic repair of childhood inguinal hernias. *Surg. Endosc.* 2004;18:957-960.
[6] Chang YT. Technical refinements in single-port laparoscopic surgery of inguinal hernia in infants and children. *Diagn. Ther. Endosc.* 2010;2010:392847.
[7] El-Gohary MA. Laparoscopic ligation of inguinal hernia in girls. *Ped. Endosurg. Innov. Techn.* 1997;1:185-188.
[8] Chang YT, Lee JY, Wang JY, Chiou CS, Chang CC. Hydrocele of the spermatic cord in infants and children: its particular characteristics. *Urology,* 2010;76:82-86.
[9] Janetschek G, Reissigl A, Bartsch G. Laparoscopic repair of pediatric hydroceles. *J. Endourol.* 1994;8:415-417.
[10] Becmeur F, Philippe P, Lemandat-Schultz A, Moog R, Grandadam S, Lieber A, Toledano D. A continuous series of 96 laparoscopic inguinal hernia repairs in children by a new technique. *Surg. Endosc.* 2004;18:1738-1741.

[11] Tsai YC, Wu CC, Yang SS. Minilaparoscopic herniorrhaphy with hernia sac transection in children and young adults: a preliminary report. *Surg. Endosc.* 2007;21:1623-1625.
[12] Giseke S, Glass M, Tapadar P, Matthyssens L, Philippe P. A true laparoscopic herniotomy in children: evaluation of long-term outcome. *J. Laparoendosc. Adv. Surg. Tech. A.* 2010;20:191-194.
[13] Tsai YC, Wu CC, Yang SS. Open versus minilaparoscopic herniorrhaphy for children: a prospective comparative trial with midterm follow-up evaluation. *Surg. Endosc.* 2010;24:21-24.
[14] Koivusalo AI, Korpela R, Wirtavuori K, Piiparinen S, Rintala RJ, Pakarinen MP. A single-blinded, randomized comparison of laparoscopic versus open hernia repair in children. *Pediatrics*, 2009;123:332-337.
[15] Schier F. Laparoscopic inguinal hernia repair-a prospective personal series of 542 children. *J. Pediatr. Surg.* 2006;41:1081-1084.
[16] Bharathi RS, Arora M, Baskaran V. How we "SEAL" internal ring in pediatric inguinal hernias. *Surg. Laparosc. Endosc. Percutan. Tech.* 2008;18:192-194.
[17] Harrison MR, Lee H, Albanese CT, Farmer DL. Subcutaneous endoscopically assisted ligation (SEAL) of the internal ring for repair of inguinal hernias in children: a novel technique. *J. Pediatr. Surg.* 2005;40:1177-1180.
[18] Ozgediz D, Roayaie K, Lee H, Nobuhara KK, Farmer DL, Bratton B, Harrison MR. Subcutaneous endoscopically assisted ligation (SEAL) of the internal ring for repair of inguinal hernias in children: report of a new technique and early results. *Surg. Endosc.* 2007;21:1327-1331.
[19] Patkowski D, Czernik J, Chrzan R, Jaworski W, Apoznański W. Percutaneous internal ring suturing: a simple minimally invasive technique for inguinal hernia repair in children. *J. Laparoendosc. Adv. Surg. Techn.* 2006;16:513-517.
[20] Chang YT, Wang JY, Lee JY, Chiou CS, Hsieh JS. One-trocar laparoscopic transperitoneal closure of inguinal hernia in children. *World J. Surg.* 2008;32:2459-2463.
[21] Chang YT, Wang JY, Lee JY, Chiou CS. A simple single-port laparoscopic-assisted technique for completely enclosing inguinal hernia in children. *Am. J. Surg.* 2009;198:e164-167.
[22] Dutta S. Early experience with single incision laparoscopic surgery: eliminating the scar from abdominal operations. *J. Pediatr. Surg.* 2009;44:1741-1745.

[23] Shen W, Ji H, Lu G, Chen Z, Li L, Zhang H, Pan J. A modified single-port technique for the minimally invasive treatment of pediatric inguinal hernias with high ligation of the vaginal process: the initial experience. *Eur. J. Pediatr.* 2010;169:1207-1212.

[24] Uchida H, Kawashima H, Goto C, Sato K, Yoshida M, Takazawa S, Iwanaka T. Inguinal hernia repair in children using single-incision laparoscopic-assisted percutaneous extraperitoneal closure. *J. Pediatr. Surg.* 2010;45:2386-2389.

[25] Riquelme M, Aranda A, Riquelme-Q M. Laparoscopic pediatric inguinal hernia repair: no ligation, just resection. *J. Laparoendosc. Adv. Surg. Tech. A.* 2010;20:77-80.

[26] Ergul E, Korukluoglu B. Peritoneal adhesions: facing the enemy. *Int. J. Surg.* 2008;6:253-260.

[27] Chan KL, Chan HY, Tam PK. Towards a near-zero recurrence rate in laparoscopic inguinal hernia repair for pediatric patients of all ages. *J. Pediatr. Surg.* 2007;42:1993-1997.

[28] P Połubinska A, Breborowicz A, Staniszewski R, Oreopoulos DG. Normal saline induces oxidative stress in peritoneal mesothelial cells. *J. Pediatr. Surg.* 2008;43:1821-1826.

[29] Oue T, Kubota A, Okuyama H, Kawahara H. Laparoscopic percutaneous extraperitoneal closure (LPEC) method for the exploration and treatment of inguinal hernia in girls. *Pediatr. Surg. Int.* 2005;21:964-968.

[30] Treef W, Schier F. Characteristics of laparoscopic inguinal hernia recurrences. *Pediatr. Surg. Int.* 2009;25:149-152.

[31] Schier F, Turial S, Hückstädt T, Klein KU, Wannik T. Laparoscopic inguinal hernia repair does not impair testicular perfusion. *J. Pediatr. Surg.* 2008;43:131-135.

[32] Lipskar AM, Soffer SZ, Glick RD, Rosen NG, Levitt MA, Hong AR. Laparoscopic inguinal hernia inversion and ligation in female children: a review of 173 consecutive cases at a single institution. *J. Pediatr. Surg.* 45:1370-1374.

In: Hernias: Types, Symptoms and Treatment ISBN: 978-1-61324-125-7
Editor: James H. Wagner © 2011 Nova Science Publishers, Inc.

Chapter 7

Incidence and Risk Factors for an Incisional Hernia after Severe Secondary Peritonitis

Pascal Jeanmonod[*], Sven Richter, Jochen Schuld, Christoph Justinger, Otto Kollmar, Martin K. Schilling and Mohammed R. Moussavian
Department of General, Visceral, Vascular and Pediatric Surgery
University of Saarland, Homburg/Saar, Germany

Abstract

Background: In patients with secondary peritonitis, infections of the abdominal cavity might render the abdominal wall susceptible to secondary complications like incisional hernia (IH). *Methods:* One hundred ninety-eight patients treated for secondary peritonitis underwent midline laparotomy.

Ninety-two surviving patients accessible to clinical follow-up were examined for the occurrence of IH and risk factors at the time of surgery or during follow-up were determined. *Results:* During a median follow-up period of 6 years 54.3% of the patients developed IHs.

---

[*]E-mail: pascal.jeanmonod@uks.eu, Phone:+49 6841 1630001

A high body mass index, coronary heart disease, intense blood loss, requirement of intraoperative or postoperative transfusions and small bowel perforation as source of peritonitis were associated with IH. *Conclusion:* IH occurs quite frequently after surgery for secondary peritonitis.

Preexisting risk factors for IH and intraoperative blood loss or requirement of blood transfusions were correlated with the development of IH. Interestingly, surgical technique was not correlated with the development of IH in this series.

Keywords: abdominal surgery, secondary peritonitis, incisional hernia.

Introduction

A midline laparotomy is the standard approach to access and eliminate the infectious source in patients with secondary peritonitis. A number of surgical strategies are available for the treatment of secondary peritonitis like (i) planned relaparotomy, (ii) on-demand relaparotomy and (iii) single high volume lavage (SHVL), with comparable postoperative mortality [1, 2]. Although goal oriented intensive care and surgical treatment and focused antibiotic strategies have improved the survival of patients with secondary peritonitis, few data are available on the long term outcome, namely, incisional hernia (IH) as a secondary complication of laparotomy. In a general surgical population 5% to 15% of patients develop incisional hernia within one year after midline laparotomy [3] and IH remains the major postoperative wound complication after open abdominal surgery. A number of factors predisposing for the development of incisional hernias have been identified such as smoking, chronic obstructive pulmonary disease (COPD), obesity, diabetes, and genetically determined collagen disorders. In patients undergoing surgical therapy for secondary peritonitis, frequent laparotomies for revision, infections of the abdominal wall, and impaired wound healing due to the systemic inflammatory response might render the abdominal wall even more susceptible to incisional hernia, compared with the general surgical population. Also, changes in capillary permeability with splanchnic edema and paralytic small bowel distension frequently contribute to elevated intra-abdominal pressure during the course of secondary peritonitis [4, 5]. High intra-abdominal pressure in turn might further impair incisional healing after laparotomy [6]. We therefore analyzed the incidence and risk factors for IH in patients with secondary peritonitis at a tertiary referral hospital.

Methods

Between January 1997 and December 2004, data from patients undergoing midline laparotomy for secondary peritonitis were collected prospectively. Patients with the following criteria were included in this analysis: age 16 to 90 years, with faecal or purulent peritonitis, caused by perforation of the gastrointestinal tract. Patients aged <16 or >90 years, those with peritonitis caused by pancreatitis, those with peritonitis due to peritoneal dialysis catheter, those with incisions other than midline incisions, and those with burst abdomen and open abdomen management without definitive closure of the abdominal fascia were excluded from the analysis. A total of 198 patients met these criteria and were analyzed retrospectively. As would be expected in patients with secondary peritonitis, bacterial wound contamination of 100% was found on microbiologic analysis in all patients (data not shown).

Surgical Technique

In our department, patients were assigned to either an on-demand, a planned, or a single high volume lavage (SHVL) strategy, as defined previously [1]. Relaparotomy was considered if there were signs of abdominal compartment syndrome with hemodynamic instability, persistent or de novo anastomotic leakage, or perforations or ischemia or necrosis of splanchnic organs.

Open abdominal management was applied in cases of abdominal compartment syndrome with subsequent impairment of pulmonary, cardiac, hepatic, or renal function. Final abdominal wall closure was achieved by a continuous fascial closure using loop suture or simple interrupted suture and surgical clips for skin closure. In cases of continuous closure, the suture length/incision length ratio was $\geq 4:1$. The running sutures were 1 cm apart and ≥ 1.5 cm from the wound edge [3, 7]. Drains, when used, were inserted through a stab wound away from the incision. A colostomy or ileostomy, when performed, was always fashioned through a separate incision. Incisional hernias were defined as protrusions of tissue or an organs through defects of the anterior abdominal wall [6, 8] causing bulges in the abdominal area of ≥ 2 cm in length and width. Hernias were classified as symptomatic or asymptomatic.

Physical Examination

Ninety-two surviving patients available for follow-up were interviewed and examined for IH and IH repair between July and November 2008 by one investigator. Length, width, color and accumulation of keloid of the scar were recorded and documented. The median follow-up period was 74 months (range, 31 – 151 months).

Data Collection

Collected data included all biographic and perioperative data as well as postoperative outcomes, including history and physical examination. Risk factors for IH, such as body mass index (BMI), patient's age, operation time, blood loss, antibiotic prophylaxis, and patient's physical status (classified according to the American Society of Anaesthesiologists) were entered prospectively into a database. Also, history and pathology of perforation and preoperative and postoperative complications during the first procedure were recorded.

Statistical Analysis

Data from all patients were entered in a database on an ISH-med SAP (St. Leon-Rot, Germany) platform. Patients were divided into two groups: patients with IHs at the time of clinical examination or histories of IH repair after peritonitis treatments and patients without signs of IHs or histories of IH repair.

Differences between the two groups were calculated by Chi-square or Fisher's exact tests for categorical variables and Mann-Whitney-U tests for continuously variables. Confidence intervals for the difference between proportions were calculated using a normal approximation of the binominal distribution using SPSS (SPSS, Inc, Chicago, IL) and SAS (SAS Institute GmbH, Heidelberg, Germany). Data are expressed as absolute numbers or as mean ±SEM.

Results

The median survival of the 198 patients with severe secondary peritonitis was 122 months. Eighty-eight patients had died, and information about IHs in the postoperative period could not be obtained. Of the remaining 110 patients, 18 patients were lost to follow-up. Ninety-two surviving patients were seen in our outpatient clinic, underwent physical examination for IH and were asked for histories of IH repair (Figure 1).

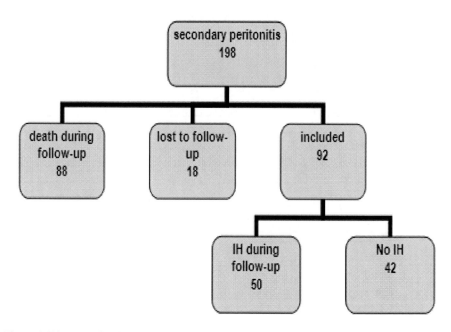

Figure 1. Diagram of 198 patients undergoing midline laparotomy after secondary peritonitis.

Demographic Data and Preoperative Risk Factors

At our institution, the incidence of IH after midline laparotomy without secondary peritonitis was 17.1% (from 2004 to 2007, 12-36 month follow-up, unpublished results), which compares favourably with data in the literature. Most patients were classified as Amercian Society of Anesthesiologists grade 3 (55 of 92 [59.8 %]) and had a number of comorbidities at the time of median laparotomy (Table 1). At that time point, patients had an average of 1.7 prior abdominal operations.

Table 1. Demographic data and history of 92 patients undergoing operation for secondary peritonitis via midline laparotomy

Patients with secondary peritonitis (n)	92
Gender (m/f) (n)	44/48
Age (years) (mean ± SEM)	53.4 ± 1.6
[1]BMI (operation day) (mean ± SEM)	26.5 ± 0.6
Comorbidities (n)	
Arterial hypertension	29
Coronary artery disease	7
Cardiac arrhythmia	6
Chronic obstructive pulmonary disease	17
Renal	13
Hepatic	9
Diabetes mellitus	17
Hyperlipidemia	16
Others	10
History of malignoma (n)	6
[2]ASA classification (1/2/3/4) (n)	2/26/55/8
Previous abdominal operations (mean ± SEM)	1.71 ± 0.15
History of perforation <24h / >24 h (n)	31/61
Site of perforation (n)	
Colon	38
Appendix	16
Anastomosis insufficiency	15
Small bowel	9
Upper gastrointestinal tract	8
Abscess	6
Fecal/Purulent	21/71
Mannheim Peritonitis Index (mean ± SEM)	22.4 ± 0.9
Planned lavage / [3]SHVL (n)	34/58
Definitive abdominal closure material (n)	
Interrupted suture	28
Continued suture	64
Total number of operations (mean ± SEM)	2.4 ± 0.2
ICU stay (d) (mean ± SEM)	6.3 ± 0.9
Hospital stay (d) (mean ± SEM)	15.9 ± 0.9
Current [1]BMI (mean ± SEM)	27.3 ± 0.6
Incision length/body length ratio (mean ± SEM)	0.13 ± 0.01

[1]body mass index (BMI), [2]American Society of Anesthesiologists (ASA), [3]single high volume lavage (SHVL), [4]ICU (intensive care unit).

The site of perforation was the colon in 41.3%, followed by perforated appendicitis (17.4%) and anastomotic leakage (16.3%). Fifty-eight of 92 patients (63.0%) were treated using single high-volume lavage.

Final closure of the abdominal cavity was performed using a single running suture in 69.6% of all patients. IHs at the time of follow-up or histories of IH repair were registered in 50 of 92 patients (54.3%). There was no gender difference between patients developing IHs or not. Preoperative BMIs were significantly higher in patients who developed IH (p=0.013). Also, coronary artery disease at the time of surgery was found as a significant risk factor for IH (p=0.012).

A multivariate analysis did not reveal any risk factor to be significant. Of 50 patients with IHs, 48% were symptomatic and 52% underwent IH repair (Table 2).

Table 2. Characteristics of IH in 50 patients

Incisional hernia	50
Symptomatic hernia at follow up n (%)	24 (48)
Hernia repair during follow up n (%)	26 (52)
Recurrent hernia	0
Recurrent hernia repair	0
Scar length (cm)	24.3 ± 1.2
Scar width (cm)	1.4 ± 0.1
Keloid n (%)	14 (28)

Intraoperative and Postoperative Risk Factors

The intraoperative data of the patients are shown in Table 3. Interestingly, surgical strategy, the number and duration of operations, and the source and severity of peritonitis measured by the Mannheim Peritonitis Index score were comparable between both groups.

Table 3. Preoperative risk factors and past medical history of 92 patients undergoing operation for secondary peritonitis via midline laparotomy

	incisional hernia		p value
	yes	no	
Patients (n)	50	42	
Gender (m/f) (n)	25/25	19/23	NS
Age (years) (mean ± SEM)	54.7 ± 1.8	51.9 ± 2.7	NS
[1]BMI (operation day) (mean ± SEM)	27.7 ± 0.8	25.2 ± 0.9	0.013
Comorbidities (n)			
Arterial hypertension	18	11	NS
Coronary artery disease	7	0	0.012
Cardiac arrhythmia	4	2	NS
Chronic obstructive pulmonary disease	10	7	NS
Renal	6	7	NS
Hepatic	7	2	NS
Diabetes mellitus	11	6	NS
Hyperlipidemia	9	7	NS
Others	5	5	NS
History of malignancy (n)	2	4	NS
[2]ASA classification (1/2/3/4) (n)	1/11/33/4	1/15/22/4	
Previous abdominal operations (mean ± SEM)	1.9 ± 0.2	1.6 ± 0.2	NS
Drugs (n)			
Cortison	9	14	NS
Other immunosuppression	4	4	NS
Statin therapy	6	4	NS
Nutritional factors (n)			
Alcohol	21	16	NS
Nicotin	23	13	NS
Fecal	12	9	NS
Purulent	38	33	
Mannheim Peritonitis Index (mean ± SEM)	23.1 ± 1.2	21.4 ± 1.4	NS
History of perforation (d) <24h (n)	16	15	NS
History of perforation (d) >24h (n)	34	27	NS
Site of perforation (n)			
Anastomosis insufficiency	7	8	NS
Colon perforation	18	20	NS
Perforated appendicitis	8	8	NS
Upper gastrointestinal perforation	5	3	NS
Small bowel perforation	8	1	NS
Abscess	4	2	NS

[1]body mass index (BMI), [2]American Society of Anesthesiologists (ASA)

However, patients who developed hernias during follow-up had more small bowel perforations (p=0.029), had higher intraoperative blood loss (p=0.014), and required more intraoperative fresh-frozen plasma transfusions (p=0.008) at the time of surgery. Of interest, the technique of final abdominal wall closure was not different between both groups.

Follow up

Postoperative transfusion of red blood cells and thrombocytes (p=0.011 and p=0.031, respectively), but not of fresh frozen plasma, was significantly different between both groups (Table 4).

Table 4. Surgical treatment in 92 patients undergoing operation for secondary peritonitis via midline laparotomy

	incisional hernia		p value
	yes	no	
Patients	50	42	
Planned lavage (n)	16	18	NS
[1]SHVL (n)	34	24	NS
Abdominal drainage (n)	36	33	NS
Operation time (min) (mean ± SEM)	111 ± 8	103 ± 6	NS
Open abdomen management (n)	19	17	NS
Abdominal closure (n)			
Interrupted suture	17	11	NS
Continued suture	33	31	NS
Total number of operations (mean ± SEM)	2.5 ± 0.3	2.3 ± 0.3	NS
Blood loss (ml) (mean ± SEM)	177 ± 67	85 ± 16	0.014
Intraoperative transfusions (mean ± SEM)			
Red blood cells	0.06 ± 0.06	0.17 ± 0.09	NS
[2]FFP	0.10 ± 0.07	0.00 ± 0.00	0.008

[1]SHVL (single high volume lavage), [2]FFP (fresh frozen plasma)

The current BMI and the ratio of incision length to body length were not different between both groups (Table 5).

Table 5. Postoperative parameters and currents physical status in 92 patients undergoing operation for secondary peritonitis via midline laparotomy

	incisional hernia		p value
	yes	no	
patients	50	42	
patients requiring transfusions (n)	12	9	NS
postoperative transfusions (mean ± SEM)			
red blood cells	1.0 ± 0.3	0.5 ± 0.2	0.011
[1]FFP	0.17 ± 0.10	0.12 ± 0.12	NS
thrombocytes	0.00 ± 0.00	0.02 ± 0.02	0.031
volume requirement (n)			
infusion volume >4.0l/24h	12	12	NS
infusion volume >6.0l/48h	16	14	NS
catecholamine therapy (n)	18	13	NS
ventilation support (n)	29	20	NS
duration of ventilation in days (mean ± SEM)	6.7 ± 1.8	4.9 ± 1.5	NS
[2]ICU stay (d) (mean ± SEM)	6.8 ± 1.3	5.6 ± 1.1	NS
hospital stay (d) (mean ± SEM)	16.4 ± 1.3	15.3 ± 1.2	NS
current [3]BMI (mean ± SEM)	28.8 ± 0.8	25.8 ± 0.8	NS
ratio incision/body length (mean ± SEM)	0.14 ± 0.01	0.12 ± 0.01	NS

[1]FFP (fresh frozen plasma), [2]ICU (intensive care unit), [3]body mass index (BMI)

Comments

The major finding of the present study is the high incidence of IH after emergency laparotomy for feculent or purulent peritonitis. In addition, we found the occurrence of IH to be independent from the surgical approach used in this series. Within 6 years after laparotomy for severe peritonitis, patients undergoing staged laparotomies did not develop more IHs than patients undergoing single laparotomies with high-volume lavage and relaparotomy on demand. Furthermore, factors commonly known as risk factors for IH, such as adipositas or cardiovascular comorbidities, were not associated with the development of IH on multivariate analysis in this series [6, 8-13].

IHs are defined as visible or palpable bulges in the former incision [9]. They occur in up to 10% of patients undergoing median laparotomies [3]. Patients with wound infections develop IHs in up to 23% or in up to 50% in patients with severe abdominal infections, as in the present and previous series [7, 13]. Not only was the incidence of IH high in this series but all hernias were classified as large hernias with an average length of 25 cm, involving the complete abdominal incision, and 50% of our patients had symptomatic IH.

The high incidence and severity of IH seen in this series can be attributed to a number of local and systemic factors [14-17]. Because of the underlying disease, all patients had infected abdominal walls, with abdominal wall edema, and at least patients with primary abdominal wound closure and a 1-stage repair might have had higher intra-abdominal pressures in the early postoperative period [18-20].

In agreement with previous studies, increased plasma C-reactive protein levels were observed in patients after the transfusion of human blood products [14]. Although the amount of mean blood loss in both groups may be negligible (177 vs. 185 ml), this parameter was significantly different between the two groups. In line with this, the difference of red blood cell and thrombocyte transfusions was significant between the two groups. A pathophysiologic explanation may be that the transfusion of human blood products causes a release of nitric oxide [15], leading to vasodilatation [16. 17] and changes in splanchnic, renal, and hepatic perfusion [18]. Together with volume replacement therapy to improve organ perfusion, this may enhance tissue edema and intra-abdominal pressure [20].This pathway could explain the high mortality and incidence of IH in patients with transfusions of human blood products in secondary peritonitis.

In addition, patients with high BMIs and the requirement for volume replacement therapy had more His [10-13]. Overall however, the severity of the underlying disease in this series, with impaired wound repair mechanisms due to the local and systemic inflammatory response might be the overriding effect over all other conventionally known factors that contribute to the development of IH [21].

Although IHs might be treated conservatively in some patients, a number of patients need to alter lifestyles or employment or undergo elective or emergency hernia repair in case of bowel strangulation or incarceration [22]. Half of our patients had undergone hernia repair at the time of follow-up, and of the remaining patients, symptomatic patients were recommended to have surgical repair.

Mesh repair is the current treatment of choice in patients with IHs, but prevention of IH should be the future strategy [21-23]. In patients with feculent or purulent peritonitis, innovative antimicrobial meshes might not only help ameliorate bacterial infection of the abdominal wall but also aid in reducing an unacceptably high incidence of IH after severe peritonitis.

The present study analyzes for the first time risk factors for the occurrence of IH after secondary peritonitis. These risk factors comprise a high BMI and a requirement for volume replacement therapy. These factors, however, are overridden by the severity of the underlying disease in this series, with impaired wound repair mechanisms due to the local and systemic inflammatory response. Therefore, future wound closure strategies need to be developed for patients with secondary peritonitis, including innovative mesh techniques, to reduce the unacceptably high incidence of IH after severe peritonitis.

References

[1] Moussavian MR, Richter S, Kollmar O, Schuld J, Schilling MK. Staged lavage versus single high-volume lavage in the treatment of feculent/purulent peritonitis: a matched pair analysis. *Langenbecks Arch. Surg.* 2009; 394: 215-220.

[2] van Ruler O, Mahler CW, Boer KR, Reuland EA, Gooszen HG, Opmeer BC, de Graaf PW, Lamme B, Gerhards MF, Steller EP, van Till JW, de Borgie CJ, Gouma DJ, Reitsma JB, Boermeester MA; Dutch Peritonitis Study Group. Comparison of on-demand vs. planned relaparotomy strategy in patients with severe peritonitis: a randomized trial. *JAMA* 2007; 298: 865-872.

[3] Bolli M, Schilling M. Incision and closure of the abdominal wall. *Chirurg,* 2006; 77: 408-413.

[4] Marx G, Pedder S, Smith L, Swaraj S, Grime S, Stockdale H, Leuwer M. Attenuation of capillary leakage by hydroxyethyl starch (130/0.42) in a porcine model of septic shock. *Crit. Care Med.* 2006; 34: 3005-3010.

[5] Marx G, Cobas Meyer M, Schuerholz T, Vangerow B, Gratz KF, Hecker H, Sümpelmann R, Rueckoldt H, Leuwer M. Hydroxyethyl starch and modified fluid gelatin maintain plasma volume in a porcine model of septic shock with capillary leakage. *Intensive Care Med.* 2002; 28: 629-635.

[6] den Hartog D, Dur AH, Tuinebreijer WE, Kreis RW. Open surgical procedures for incisional hernias. *Cochrane Database Syst. Rev.* 2008; 3: Review.

[7] Justinger C, Moussavian MR, Schlueter C, Kopp B, Kollmar O, Schilling MK. Antibiotic coating of abdominal closure sutures and wound infection. *Surgery,* 2009; 145, 330-334.
[8] Höer J, Lawong G, Klinge U, Schumpelick V. Factors influencing the development of incisional hernia. A retrospective study of 2,983 laparotomy patients over a period of 10 years. *Chirurg,* 2002; 73: 474-480.
[9] Jargon D, Friebe V, Hopt UT, Obermaier R. Risk Factors and Prevention of Incisional Hernia - What is Evidence-Based? *Zentralbl. Chir.* 2008; 133: 453-457.
[10] Mäkelä JT, Kiviniemi H, Juvonen T, Laitinen S. Factors influencing wound dehiscence after midline laparotomy. *Am. J. Surg.* 1995; 170: 387-390.
[11] Riou JP, Cohen JR, Johnson H Jr. Factors influencing wound dehiscence. *Am. J. Surg.* 1992; 163: 324-330.
[12] Israelsson LA, Jonsson T. Incisional hernia after midline laparotomy: a prospective study. *Eur. J. Surg.* 1996; 162: 125-129.
[13] Marwah S, Marwah N, Singh M, Kapoor A, Karwasra RK. Addition of rectus sheath relaxation incisions to emergency midline laparotomy for peritonitis to prevent fascial dehiscence. *World J. Surg.* 2005; 29: 235-239.
[14] Fransen E, Maessen J, Dentener M, Senden N, Buurman W. Impact of blood transfusions on inflammatory mediator release in patients undergoing cardiac surgery. *Chest* 1999; 116: 1233-1239.
[15] Wallis JP. Nitric oxide and blood: a review. *Transfus Med.* 2005;15:1-11.
[16] Jia L, Bonaventura C, Bonaventura J, Stamler JS. S-nitrosohaemoglobin: a dynamic activity of blood involved in vascular control. *Nature,* 1996; 380: 221-226.
[17] Crawford JH, White CR, Patel RP. Vasoactivity of S-nitrosohemoglobin: role of oxygen, heme, and NO oxidation states. *Blood* 2003; 101: 4408-4415.
[18] Diebel LN, Wilson RF, Dulchavsky SA, Saxe J. Effect of increased intra-abdominal pressure on hepatic arterial, portal venous, and hepatic microcirculatory blood flow. *J. Trauma,* 1992; 33: 279-282.
[19] Vincent JL, De Backer D. Microvascular dysfunction as a cause of organ dysfunction in severe sepsis. *Crit. Care* 2005; 9: 9-12.
[20] Höer J, Klinge U, Anurov M, Titkova S, Oettinger A, Schumpelick V. Tension banding closure of laparotomies: results of an experimental study in dogs. *Langenbecks Arch. Surg* 2002; 387: 309-314.
[21] Cassar K, Munro A. Surgical treatment of incisional hernia *Br. J. Surg.* 2002;89(5):534-45.

[22] Venclauskas L, Silanskaite J, Kanisauskaite J, Kiudelis M. Long-term results of incisional hernia treatment. *Medicina* (Kaunas). 2007;43(11):855-60.

[23] Korenkov M, Paul A, Sauerland S, Neugebauer E, Arndt M, Chevrel JP, Corcione F, Fingerhut A, Flament JB, Kux M, Matzinger A, Myrvold HE, Rath AM, Simmermacher RK. Classification and surgical treatment of incisional hernia. Results of an experts' meeting. *Langenbecks Arch. Surg.* 2001 Feb;386(1):65-73.

In: Hernias: Types, Symptoms and Treatment ISBN: 978-1-61324-125-7
Editor: James H. Wagner © 2011 Nova Science Publishers, Inc.

Chapter 8

Surgical Approach to Umbilical Hernias: Then and Now

Igor Belyansky, Victor B. Tsirline, David A. Klima, Ronald F. Sing, and B. Todd Heniford[*]

Division of Gastrointestinal and Minimally Invasive Surgery, Carolinas Laparoscopic and Advanced Surgery Program, Carolinas Medical Center, Charlotte, North Carolina, USA

Abstract

Congenital umbilical hernia is the most common abdominal wall defect in children. Most surgeons agree to pursue nonoperative management before age 5 unless the hernia is symptomatic, incarcerated or strangulated. Umbilical hernias in adults comprise only 6% of all abdominal wall hernias, with over 90% of these defects being acquired, presenting in the fifth or sixth decades of life. Etiologies are multifactorial. Typical adult umbilical hernia patients include: those with a history of prostatic hypertrophy, chronic obstructive pulmonary disease (COPD), constipation, hepatic cirrhosis with ascites, morbid obesity and multiparous women. The umbilical hernia sack may include omentum, small bowel and colon. Incarceration and strangulation of abdominal viscera in umbilical hernias is 14-fold more likely

---

[*] Address correspondence to: B. Todd Heniford, MD, 1025 Morehead Medical Drive, Suit 300, Charlotte, NC 28204, Phone (704) 355-3168, Fax (704) 355-4117, Email: todd.heniford@carolinashealthcare.org

in adults than in children. Adult umbilical hernias rarely resolve spontaneously, and strong consideration should be given to prompt repair because of its association with increased morbidity and mortality. Traditionally, umbilical hernia repair is an open procedure, but recently several laparoscopic or laparoscopic-assisted approaches have been described. The use of mesh has drastically changed the surgical approach to hernia repair, demonstrating a dramatic decrease in hernia recurrence rates. But the use of mesh produces its own unique complications: rarely patients can present with bowel obstruction due to adhesions to the mesh, hernia recurrence can occur as a result of mesh contraction, and cases of complete mesh migration into small bowel have been reported. Postoperative pain is usually well controlled. Interestingly, when laparoscopic approach is used, fixation of mesh with transabdominal sutures is a unique source of prolonged postoperative pain. Following simple suture repair or Mayo repair, recurrence rates range from 11% to 54%. The use of mesh has lowered the recurrence rate to 1%. The lower recurrence rate with mesh is most likely a result of tension-free repair.

Pediatric Umbilical Hernia

Congenital umbilical hernias are the most common abdominal wall defects observed in children [1]. The incidence of this defect has been reported as high as 23% in a recent prospective study of African children [2]. Umbilical hernias are frequently seen in newborns, especially in premature infants of African American decent [3]. Many approaches to treat this common problem have been described in the literature over the last century ranging from early surgical intervention to application of adhesive tape to approximate the skin over the hernia site [4]. By the 1960s, many of these practices were abandoned based on the observation that umbilical hernias in premature infants tend to resolve spontaneously [4]. Soon after birth, a patent umbilical ring contracts by receiving additional reinforcement from the lateral umbilical ligament, the round ligament and the urachus [3]. A one centimeter (cm) umbilical defect has been shown to close spontaneously in 95% of the cases within the first 5 years of life, with most undergoing spontaneous closure in the first 3 years of life [3-6].

Because of the high rate of spontaneous closure of congenital umbilical hernias, most surgeons opt for nonoperative management before age 5 unless the hernia is symptomatic, incarcerated or strangulated [4, 6]. Interestingly, incarceration is rare in newborns, thus it is safe to observe children with this defect, and prophylactic repair of small hernias is not justified [6, 7]. Defects larger than 1 cm in diameter are less likely to close spontaneously before school age and need to be closely followed, as future surgical intervention may be required [6]. Although spontaneous defect closure may occur at up to 14 years of age [2], surgical repair is recommended just before starting school, since the rate on incarceration is high in this age group [5].

Adult Umbilical Hernia

Introduction and Indications

Umbilical and para-umbilical hernias are the two most common types of spontaneous adult hernias and account for 10% of all primary abdominal wall hernias [8]. In the adult population, 90% of umbilical hernias are acquired and represent the indirect herniation through the umbilical canal [3, 9, 10]. The acquired types of umbilical hernias are typically seen in individuals in their fifth or sixth decade of life [3, 9-12]. Women are three times as likely to have an umbilical hernia as men and have higher morbidity and mortality rates associated with these [3, 9, 12, 13].

The umbilical canal has four borders: the umbilical fascia posteriorly, the linea alba anteriorly, and the medial edges of the rectus sheath on each side [3]. Etiologies of acquired umbilical hernia may be multifactorial, but all are related to chronic elevation in intra-abdominal pressure causing a gradual yielding of scar tissue that closes the umbilical ring, resulting in fascial weakness at the umbilical area [3, 9]. Typical adult umbilical hernia patients include: those with a history of prostatic hypertrophy, COPD, constipation, hepatic cirrhosis with ascites, morbid obesity and multiparous women [3, 9, 14].

The World Health Organization estimates that there will be 2.3 billion overweight adults and more than 700 million obese adults in 2015 [15]. The high prevalence of obesity is associated with an increased incidence of diverse diseases, hypertension, hypercholestronemia, type 2 *diabetes* mellitus, obstructive sleep apnea, asthma, cardiovascular disease, degenerative joint disease, diverse types of cancer, hernias and depression [15]. With the epidemic of morbid obesity on the rise, the number of abdominal wall hernias performed yearly is also increasing [15, 16]. More than ever, surgeons are now faced with operating on patients with multiple morbidities, although the most optimal surgical approach to umbilical hernia remains undetermined.

Adult umbilical hernias rarely resolve spontaneously, and strong consideration should be given to prompt repair because of its association with increased morbidity and mortality [13, 17]. The umbilical hernia sack may include omentum, small bowel and colon [9]. Hernia sizes vary, but large hernias with a narrow fascial neck are associated with higher risk of strangulation [14]. Incarceration and strangulation of abdominal viscera in umbilical hernias is 14-fold more likely in adults than in children [9]. When an elective surgical procedure is not scheduled in a timely fashion, umbilical hernias can significantly increase in size [14] or can lead to abdominal viscera incarceration. Massive hernias can give rise to dystrophic skin ulcerations, as a consequence effecting the decision for synthetic mesh placement. These large hernias can cause chronic abdominal and back pain and respiratory complications due to diaphragmatic dysfunction [14]. Furthermore, continued loss of abdominal domain can further complicate a repair. Incarcerated external hernias are the second most common cause of small intestinal obstruction, occur 5% of the time, require an emergent operative exploration, and occur in a significantly higher proportion of women [13]. Thirteen percent of incarcerated abdominal wall hernias are umbilical [10], with 20% of these requiring nonviable bowel resection due to delay in diagnosis [10].

A majority of individuals with umbilical hernia present as outpatients to a physician's office, most frequently complaining of pain and discomfort at the site of the fascial defect. Patients may describe a history of a bulge at the site of fascial defect that reduces spontaneously or with gentle assistance while lying down. Contrary to this, patients with incarceration present emergently. Kulah et al. reported the presentations and outcomes of a large series of patients with incarcerated abdominal hernias, and the most common presentation was a mass in the abdominal wall and localized pain [13]. Thirty-nine percent of their patients had the diagnosis of strangulation, and 63% had a bowel obstruction, with the large number of incarcerations related to delay in elective repair [13]. Prompt diagnosis is critical, since operative delay is associated with high morbidity and mortality rates [13-15, 18]. In adults, the differential diagnosis of an umbilical mass also includes an omphalomesenteric duct, urachal cyst, or Sister Mary Joseph's node and should be investigated when clinically applicable [9]. Along with history and physical, judicious use of imaging modalities such as computer tomography, colonoscopy and ultrasonography is recommended in the adult population [3].

General Operative Principles and Issues

In 1901, William J. Mayo read his work before the American Surgical Association, titled An Operation for the Radical Cure of Umbilical Hernia, in which he described the "vest over pants" approach of imbricating the edges of the fascial defect onto themselves [19]. This novel technique has revolutionized the field of hernia surgery, with many surgeons adapting this method of repair for the majority of the 20th century [3, 11]. This approach requires extensive fascial dissection and overlapping [3, 19, 20]. When addressing very large umbilical hernias, the fascial edges are difficult to bring together in a tension-free manner [3, 21, 22]. Since the Mayo repair incorporates a fascial overlap, sutures can cause tension on the tissues, increasing the risk of tissue ischemia and suture cut-through [14]. Frequently, the early postoperative period is complicated by significant pain, flap devascularization, and a high incidence of wound infections [20]. Furthermore, bringing the edges of the defect together may result in the decrease of abdominal domain causing elevated intra-abdominal pressure [20], leading to surgical repair failure. This is especially true when dealing with a large hernia defect.

The size of the hernia defect [14, 20] and body mass index [12] have been shown in multiple studies to be predictive of repair failure. Although the Mayo technique had a dramatic effect on reduction of hernia recurrence rates in the early 20th century, these rates are still high by present standards [3, 8, 19]. Umbilical hernia recurrence rates for primary tissue and Mayo repairs vary in the literature and range from 11% to 54% [3, 8, 14]. The importance of an anatomic repair without tension and without an artificial enlargement of the defect predict low recurrence rates [3]. Luijendijk et al. showed that primary hernia repairs, with defects of <3 cm, 3 to 6 cm, >6 to 12 cm, and >12 cm had recurrence rates of 31%, 44%, 73%, and 78%, respectively [14].

Pros and Cons of Mesh Repair

In 1955, the introduction of polypropylene mesh to strengthen a hernia repair has dramatically improved abdominal hernia recurrence outcomes [23]. For primary umbilical defects in adults, the only randomized clinical trial to date was performed by Arroyo et al. who compared suture and mesh repairs to establish a standard technique for treatment [11]. In this trial, the hernia sac was kept intact and reduced into the intra-abdominal cavity. Depending on the randomly assigned group, this was followed by use of polypropylene prosthesis or use of sutures to close the defect primarily [11]. In the group treated with prostheses, a mesh plug was used for defects smaller than 3 cm, and a mesh sheet was placed in the preperitoneal plane for larger defects [11]. This study showed a 1% recurrence rate with mesh and 11% without mesh [11] and established that the associated morbidity (infection, seroma, and hematoma) was not increased over that of suture repair [11]. In a similar study, Aslani et al. also demonstrated that the wound complication rates are similar between the primary repair and mesh repair, with a ten-fold decrease in the recurrence rate in the mesh group [8].

When to use mesh for umbilical hernia repair is still a subject of some controversy among surgeons. Although Arroyo et al. showed that the risk of postoperative complications does not increase when using prosthetics, surgeons are still reluctant to use mesh due to the additional cost associated with it as well as the perceived increase in infection rate [8]. Indeed, the use of prosthetic implants may be a "double edged sword", with the risk of seeding the mesh with microorganisms intraoperatively [24], resulting in a devastating mesh infection that often requires multiple operations to remove the source and fix the defect that is left behind [25-28]. As a matter of fact, besides the technical failure to create a tension-free repair, wound infection is the most important factor contributing to the development of a hernia recurrence [14]. In a clean case, when a prosthesis is used for hernia repair along with a preoperative prophylactic dose of an antibiotic, the infection rate is 1% to 2% [29, 30].

It is widely accepted that a tension-free approach is the key to a durable and robust hernia repair [3, 21, 22]. While performing a primary closure, tension is a factor of the defect size. When dealing with a large defect, attempts to bring the edges of the fascia together result in greater tension than when dealing with a smaller defect. The introduction of mesh to hernia repair has enabled surgeons to perform a tension-free repair by simply bridging the defect with a piece of prosthetic material. Many studies have attempted to determine the defect size below which the risks of mesh use outweigh the benefits of a tension-free repair. Unfortunately, this is still debated, with various surgical literature sources making different recommendations. Luijendijk et al. demonstrated that umbilical hernias smaller than 4 cm had a significantly lower recurrence rates [14], making a recommendation to use mesh for all defect sizes larger than 6 cm [14]. Publications by Halm et al. and Roberts et al. recommend the use of prostheses for defects greater than 3 cm [10, 20]. Furthermore, mesh use should also be considered in patents with comorbidities such as morbid obesity, prostatic hypertrophy, COPD, constipation, and liver cirrhosis with ascites, because these disease processes lead to chronically elevated intra-abdominal pressure [12, 31]. Steroids are also a unique patient risk factor that was shown to delay wound healing for small and large hernias [14], mesh use in these patients should be strongly considered regardless of the defect size. Finally, in recurrent hernia cases, mesh should be the first choice for the repair [8].

Some surgeons may still be reluctant to use mesh repair due to the additional cost associated with it. When calculating the cost of umbilical hernia repair without mesh, one must account for the cost of re-operation for hernia recurrence, which occurs 11% to 54% [3, 8, 14] of the time. By such estimates the ultimate cost of a primary umbilical hernia repair is actually higher than when mesh is used [8, 32]. Surgeons should consider all factors in deciding the appropriate type of repair based on the patient's medical condition. Although the benefits of mesh use in adult umbilical hernia repair are clear, with much lower recurrence rates compared with simple or Mayo repairs [8, 11, 14], synthetic mesh reinforcement is strongly discouraged in a contaminated field [32], and other options should be considered in this situation. The choices include simple closure or Mayo repairs for smaller defects, but when dealing with very large defects, the use of bioprosthetic materials must be strongly considered [33]. Component separation is beyond the scope of this chapter and will not be discussed here.

Biologic meshes have been developed and promoted for use in contaminated fields but are not without shortcomings. Unlike their synthetic counterparts, biosynthetics have better integration properties with the native tissue [34]. Overall, biologic meshes may allow the host to eradicate low bacterial loads of up to 10^4 CFU but become rapidly integrated into the tissues, losing their tensile strength. However, moderate infection challenges (10^6 CFU) of the biologic mesh lead to infection, as reflected by the final bacterial counts, as do synthetic implants [35, 36]. When compared with a primary repair in a clean field, the biologic reinforcement approach has a lower recurrence rate of 5% [32]. Biomaterials are significantly more expensive and probably without the long-term efficacy of synthetic materials; their use should be limited to appropriate clinical situations. Little long-term follow-up data exist to support their use in clean cases of umbilical hernia repair or any clean hernia repair. Current data indicate that adult umbilical hernias repaired with synthetic prostheses [3, 8, 11, 14] have lower recurrence rates than hernias repaired with bioprosthetics [32].

Surgical Innovations

The advent of laparoscopic surgery has popularized a minimally invasive approach to abdominal wall hernia repair. This method delivers full intra-abdominal access through several small incisions and enables the surgeon to concomitantly look prior to surgery for any other abdominal defects that may have been missed. This unique approach results in improved cosmesis and possibly in enhanced long-term patient satisfaction [37, 38]. Multiple studies have demonstrated that the laparoscopic approach is associated with a reduction in wound-related complications [18, 20, 37], most likely due to less subcutaneous dissection than is required during an open approach. Although there is evidence that patients may return to the activities of daily living sooner [37], studies looking at postoperative pain in patients that have undergone laparoscopic umbilical or ventral hernia repairs show variable results [20, 39, 40]. Laparoscopy carries additional advantages for patients at high risk for recurrence such as the morbidly obese and those with large defects [20].

Variations of the minimally invasive technique appear throughout the literature, with some described in greater detail in the Surgical Procedures section of this chapter. The general principle of a laparoscopic approach to umbilical hernias is based on the concept of a tension-free hernia repair made by bridging the defect with an intraperitoneally placed prosthesis [39, 41]. In order to do this, a generous (5 cm) circumferential overlap of the fascia with prosthetic material must be performed [39, 41]. The mesh is secured in place with a combination of trans-fascial sutures and laparoscopically placed tacks. Long-term recurrence rates are similar to those seen in open tension-free repair [37, 39, 41-43].

Preoperative Planning

Over 95% of umbilical defects are repaired as an elective procedure, and preoperative medical assessment is necessary. In patients with active respiratory infections, chronic cough, urinary tract infections, or skin infection around the surgical site, elective repair may need to be delayed until further work-up is completed and the infectious process is treated. Obviously, incarceration and/or strangulation of abdominal viscera in the hernia defect makes this procedure emergent.

Severe pulmonary disease and cardiomyopathy are a relative contraindication to laparoscopic surgery. Once the abdomen is insufflated, the decision to proceed with laparoscopy depends on how the patient tolerates elevated intraabdominal pressure. Furthermore, the surgeon should be ready to convert to an open repair in a case where elevated intraabdominal pressure adversely affects the cardiopulmonary system.

In some cases, preoperative imaging may aid in detecting visceral herniation, enabling the necessary planning. Advanced imaging may also assist in ruling out differential diagnoses, such as: omphalomesenteric duct, urachal cyst or Sister Mary Joseph's node. In cases where bowel manipulation or resection is anticipated, the use of mechanical bowel prep may be prudent.

The surgery may be performed under general, spinal or local anesthesia. General anesthesia is a method of choice in children and can be used in adults unless medically contraindicated. Spinal anesthesia may be optimal for abdominal musculature relaxation. Patient should be non-per-os after midnight before surgery.

Special Cases

Umbilical Hernia in Pregnant Patients

Pregnant patients undergo a number of unique physiological changes that induce body collagen remodeling. Relaxin is a hormone that is responsible for these changes. It is primarily produced by the corpus luteum and attains the highest levels during pregnancy [44]. This hormone plays an important role in softening of the tissues of the birth canal, thus preparing the mother's body for child delivery [44, 45]. The elevated levels of relaxin predispose women to hernia formation during pregnancy [46], specifically umbilical hernias. The literature on this subject is limited, but there is general consensus that asymptomatic hernia defects can be followed until after delivery [46, 47]. Surgical intervention is deferred to avoid exposing the fetus to general anesthesia, especially in the first trimester [46, 47]. Anesthesia related uterine irritability followed by premature labor is the primary concern during the third trimester [46, 47].

Interestingly, very low rates of incarceration are seen during pregnancy, probably as a result of the expanding uterus that displaces bowel and omentum up and out of the pelvis [47]. Visceral strangulation during pregnancy is a surgical emergency. Incarceration also demands a surgical intervention, since there is concern that the enlarging uterus may cause strangulation resulting in a devastating outcome to the mother and the fetus [46, 47].

Timing of elective repair after delivery is debated, with some arguing that umbilical hernia defects may be addressed when performing a caesarian section [46]. The opponents to early repair argue that relaxin levels remain elevated in the early port-partum period, predisposing to a higher rate of hernia recurrence [44, 45, 47]. All post-partum females with an umbilical hernia should be evaluated by a surgeon and promptly scheduled for an elective repair.

Umbilical Hernia in Cirrhotic Patients

It has been shown that chronically elevated intra-abdominal pressure is related to the development of abdominal wall hernias [3, 9, 14]. Umbilical hernias in patients with severe liver disease are common and are attributed to the combination of chronically elevated intra-abdominal pressure and weakness of the abdominal fascia [48, 49], which together cause gradual yielding of the scar tissue around the umbilical ring. Cirrhotic patients pose a unique challenge to the hernia surgeon and the optimal management is not clearly defined in the current literature [49, 50].

Traditionally, hernia repair in the presence of advanced liver disease has resulted in high morbidity and mortality [49]. This has prompted many surgeons to avoid elective repair and to operate only when the hernia complications develop [49]. Typical complications of conservative management include skin ulceration and leakage of the ascitic fluid that may result in bacterial peritonitis and serious morbidity [49, 51]. Nonoperative management of ruptured hernias with antibiotics and dressing changes has been shown to result in mortality rates of 60% to 88% [49]. Other common complications include incarceration and strangulation of the omentum or abdominal viscera. These emergent conditions demand a surgical intervention, which is associated with a mortality rate of 14% [49].

Recent literature on this subject demonstrates that an elective repair is the safest choice, as it decreases complication and mortality rates associated with conservative management [49, 51]. Ascites must be medically optimized prior to an elective umbilical hernia repair [51], as elevated intra-abdominal pressure from ascites is associated with a 30% morbidity, 5% mortality and 73% hernia recurrence [3, 49, 51, 52]. However, the control of ascites may be challenging and not always possible with diuretics and paracentesis [51]. In the case of refractory ascites, strong consideration should be given to portal decompression by a transjugular intrahepatic portosystemic shunt (TIPS) [51]. Once control of ascites is established, umbilical hernia repair is associated with a morbidity rate of 15%, mortality of 0% and recurrence of 17% [49, 51, 52].

There are several case reports of fulminant liver failure requiring emergent transplant following an umbilical hernia repair, where a patent umbilical vein was inadvertently ligated [53, 54]. For that reason, part of the preoperative workup should include an abdominal computed tomography (CT) or an abdominal Doppler ultrasound to screen for a re-opened umbilical vein that may serve as a critical conduit for portal-to-systemic blood outflow [48, 50]. If a patent umbilical vein is identified, the surgeon must proceed with caution to avoid injury to this structure, which can result in a poor patient outcome.

Patients with advanced liver disease often suffer from severe malnutrition, a condition that naturally progresses to muscle wasting and weakness in the abdominal fascia [48, 50]; these factors result in impaired wound healing, and the use of a prosthetic reinforcement becomes paramount. Ammar performed a prospective randomized study in cirrhotic patients comparing umbilical hernia repair with mesh to primary closure with sutures, which demonstrated significantly lower recurrence rates of 2.7% in the mesh group compared with 14.2% for primary repair ($p<0.05$) [50]. No mesh exposure or fistulae were observed, and there were no statistical differences in the complication rates (hematoma, seroma, ascitic fluid leakage, surgical site infection) between the groups [50].

Laparoscopy is a relative contraindication in patients with portal hypertension [55], since the elevated intra-abdominal pressure from the pneumoperitoneum may impede collateral portal outflow in a cirrhotic patient and cause ischemia-reperfusion injury to the internal organs such as liver and kidney [56]. On the other hand, laparoscopy carries potential benefits in cirrhotic patients [51, 56-58], as this minimally invasive approach has been associated with a decrease in wound infections and postoperative recovery time [18, 20, 37]. To prevent end-organ injury, surgeons who perform laparoscopy on a cirrhotic patient should strongly consider keeping the insufflation pressure below 10 mm Hg [56-58], so as not to exceed the portal venous pressure.

Surgical Procedures

Open Umbilical Hernia Repair Positioning

The patient is placed in supine position with both arms out.

Open Umbilical Hernia Repair

A wide surgical prep of the skin is performed with either Betadine™ or chlorhexidine. Traditionally a curved infraumbilical or supraumbilical incision is made. Dissection is carried out to the umbilical stalk to identify the defect. Blunt dissection is performed around the hernia sac circumferentially. Sharp dissection is used to separate the distal portion of the sac from the dermis of the umbilicus, creating an umbilical skin flap. The sac may be entered under direct visualization and appropriate adhesiolysis should be performed to facilitate reduction of its contents back into the abdomen. Excess sac may be excised. The authors recommend closing the peritoneal defect with 3-0 absorbable sutures. Alternatively, the hernia sac with its contents may be reduced in its entirety.

Musculoaponeurotic fascia must be cleared 3 cm from the edge of the defect in all directions. If the defect is less than 3 cm, it may be closed primarily with #0 nonabsorbable sutures (polypropylene or polytetrafluoroethylene). An alternative to simple suture closure is the Mayo technique, where the fascial edges of the defect are imbricated onto itself. The doubling of fascia is performed with nonabsorbable mattress suture, beginning from 3 cm from the margin of overlay fascia [3, 19]. This is followed by fixation of the free margin of the overlay to the surface of the abdominal fascia using a nonabsorbable suture [3, 19]. In a case where there is too much tension on the repair and the defect is closed in a vertical fashion, relaxing incisions on anterior rectus sheath can be performed to relieve the tension [3]. The authors advocate the use of Mayo repair technique when mesh is not an option.

For defects larger than 3 cm, the use of mesh has been shown to be beneficial in reducing hernia recurrence from 11% to 1% [11, 59]. A variety of prosthetic material is commercially available for umbilical hernia repairs. There are five possible locations of mesh placement [8, 60]:

1. Preaponeurotic space – Onlay mesh technique is used to reinforce the primary closure of a hernia defect by attaching the prosthesis to the anterior abdominal fascia, thus overlying the closed defect.
2. Fascial layer – This is known as a bridging technique. The prosthesis is attached to the edges of the hernia defect without performing primary closure.
3. Retromuscular prefascial space – The surgeon develops a plane between the rectus muscle and posterior rectus sheath. Consequently, mesh is placed in the developed space, thus overlapping the hernia defect.
4. Preperitoneal space – In this technique, a plane between the posterior fascia and the peritoneum is carefully developed using blunt dissection. This is followed by mesh placement in the developed space, thus overlapping the fascial defect.
5. Intraperitoneal space - The surgeon places the mesh intra-abdominally in the underlay fashion.

Irrespective of the choice of prosthesis, the authors recommend preperitoneal underlay placement of the mesh. The preperitoneal plane is relatively avascular, and the peritoneum serves as a native tissue barrier between the prosthetic mesh and the abdominal viscera. The prosthetic material should be appropriately sized to afford a 5-cm fascial overlap beyond the edge of the defect in all directions. Primary closure of the defect should be performed if it can be accomplished in a relatively tension-free manner. Thus, if the patient develops a superficial wound infection, the fascia overlying the mesh may prevent the spread of bacteria onto the prosthesis.

After appropriate hemostasis is achieved, a 3.0 absorbable suture can be used to tack the umbilical dermis down to the fascia and restore the natural concavity of the umbilicus. Several interrupted 3.0 absorbable sutures can be used in that fashion to minimize the dead space around the umbilical stalk thus limiting the space for seroma formation and hematoma collection. Skin is closed with a running 4.0 absorbable subcuticular suture.

"Scarless" Open Umbilical Hernia Repair

Instead of making an infraumbilical or supraumbilical incision, a vertical skin incision is made directly through the umbilicus. Sharp dissection is used to separate the distal portion of the hernia sac from the umbilical dermis. Bilateral umbilical skin flaps are raised. Circumferential blunt and sharp dissection is carried through the subcutaneous fat to the level of the fascial defect exposing the hernia sac in entirety. The treatment of sac and fascial defect is described above.

Umbilical inversion is recreated by using two interrupted 4.0 absorbable sutures placed across the midline approximating the skin down to the fascia. Another 4.0 absorbable suture is used to close the skin in a running subcuticular fashion. When fully healed, the surgical scar is not visible [9].

Laparoscopic Umbilical Hernia Repair

The patient is placed in a supine position with the upper extremities tucked at the sides. The patient must be secured to the operating table for steep tilting that may be necessary for gravity-assisted retraction to provide optimal exposure. A wide surgical prep of the skin is performed with either Betadine™ or chlorhexidine. Placement of a nasogastric tube and a urine catheter may be necessary depending on the intraoperative port placement. The authors prefer to use a Veress needle through the left upper quadrant to establish pneumoperitoneum. A scalpel is used to make a 5-mm incision in the left upper quadrant; the Veress needle is inserted, and the abdomen is insufflated with CO_2 to 14 mm Hg. Alternatives to the Veress needle insufflation include a Hassan technique or use of a Visiport™ (Ethicon, Cincinnati, OH USA).

A 5-mm trocar is then placed through the incision. A 45-degree angled scope is inserted to examine the intra-abdominal domain. Special attention should be paid to make sure that there are no other abdominal wall defects. Two additional 5-mm trocars are placed under direct visualization, one in the left lower quadrant taking care not to injure the left inferior epigastric vessels and one in the left flank. Triangulation of the work space is thus achieved.

Alternatively, a laparoscopic umbilical hernia repair can be performed with only two 5-mm ports; one camera port and one working port. This decision should be made intraoperatively and depends on the amount of intra-abdominal adhesions and the difficulty of reducing the hernia contents to the proper anatomic location. Introduction of one or two additional 5-mm ports has no adverse effects on postoperative pain, wound complications or cosmesis, and surgeons should not hesitate to place additional working ports.

The assistant holds the camera inserted through the lateral (middle) port. Soft bowel graspers are used to reduce the hernia contents to their proper anatomic location. Sharp dissection with laparoscopic scissors may be required to take down the avascular distal attachments of the hernia sac contents. Once the hernia contents are reduced, the defect size should be estimated. This can be achieved by using the tip of a soft bowel grasper or by transilluminating the defect and marking it out with spinal needles and measuring the dimensions of the markings on the abdominal surface.

Mesh size should be chosen to afford a 5-cm fascial overlap around the defect. Once the mesh is appropriately sized, four #0 non-absorbable (multifilament braided polyester) sutures are placed around the perimeter of the mesh. The prosthesis is then rolled in a "cigar" fashion, keeping in mind its orientation, and loaded onto a laparoscopic heavy grasper. There are several ways to introduce mesh into the abdominal cavity. The authors prefer to remove a working 5-mm trocar and gently dilate the tract with a surgical clamp. The heavy laparoscopic grasper with mesh is introduced intracorporeally through the dilated tract with a twisting motion on the grasper while advancing through subcutaneous and fascial layers. The 5-mm port is then replaced. Alternatively, a 5-mm port can be replaced with a 12-mm port, and mesh can be introduced through the larger trocar.

The mesh is unfolded keeping appropriate orientation. A suture passer is inserted through the previously marked sites on the abdominal surface and used to bring out the ends of the sutures tied to the corners of the mesh, one suture at a time. Gentle traction is applied to the sutures to make sure that the mesh is not too loose or under too much tension. The sutures are then tied down resulting in transfascial fixation of the mesh corners. A laparoscopic tacking device is then used to fix the mesh to the abdominal wall at approximately 1 cm increments and 0.5 cm from the edge of the mesh. Various brands of tackers and configuration of tacks are available, including permanent or absorbable tacks.

The abdomen is then deflated under direct visualization while ensuring that the mesh preserves its integrity and remains tension-free. All of the trocars are removed under direct visualization. The skin is closed with 4-0 absorbable sutures. When a 12-mm trocar is used, a fascial closure device should be used to close the defect with #0 permanent or long-term absorbable suture.

Postoperative Management

Most elective umbilical hernia repairs, open and laparoscopic, are outpatient procedures. Depending on the comorbidities, a patient may need postoperative observation. Pain is usually well controlled with oral pain medications. Patients may resume regular activity as tolerated immediately after surgery, although heavy lifting is discouraged until after the first postoperative visit. Some surgeons advise their patients to wear elastic abdominal binders in the early postoperative period, which may be of some benefit for comfort; however, no randomized trials have shown a difference in surgical outcomes with use of abdominal binders [61].

Complications

The umbilical hernia repair may be complicated by a hematoma, seroma formation or a local wound infection. The rates of these complications are similar to other clean procedures and have been reported to be 4.5% when mesh is used [8, 11, 62]. The use of mesh has drastically changed the surgical approach to the umbilical hernia repair, specifically reducing umbilical hernia recurrence to 1% compared with 11% when the Mayo repair was used [8, 11, 59]. But the use of mesh has its own unique complications. In their experience with mesh devices for intraperitoneal umbilical hernia repair, Muysoms et al. reported that patients may present with bowel obstruction due to adhesions to the mesh, hernia recurrence can occur due to mesh contraction and, in several case reports, mesh migration into the bowel required an emergent operation [31].

When the laparoscopic approach is used, fixation of the mesh with transfascial sutures is a unique source of prolonged postoperative pain. Carbonell et al. reported 23% of patients had transabdominal suture site pain [40]. This problem was successfully addressed with injection of a local anesthetic at the level of abdominal musculature [40].

Elective procedures have a mortality rate of 0 to 0.02% for patients less than 60 years of age, and 0.5% for those older than 60 [18]. For an emergent hernia operation, the mortality is higher, ranging from 0.5% to 15% [14, 18]. Global morbidity of an incarcerated external hernia ranges from 19% to 46%, with the major morbidity (pulmonary, cardiac, renal, or digestive disease) ranging between 10% and 15% [15]. The main factors influencing morbidity and mortality are: age (>60), hernias of more than 10 years in evolution, delayed hospitalization (after more than 48 hours of symptoms), concomitant disease, American Society of Anesthesiologists (ASA) III or IV class and viability of entrapped bowel [13, 15].

The probability of death is increased in patients with age over 70 years, higher ASA class, and associated intestinal resection [18]. The emergency surgical procedure mortality rate is between 3% and 13% and has remained unchanged in the last 15 years [14, 15, 18]. The most common causes of death are pneumonia and respiratory failure [18]. Resection of nonviable bowel has been shown to be associated with a 75% mortality rate [18].

Conclusion

The repair of an umbilical hernia defect can include a variety of methods and can be performed either using an open or laparoscopic approach. The decision to use a traditional open or laparoscopic method must be based on the hernia size, patient factors, and the surgeon's experience and training. When using the open approach, the authors favor the use of mesh for umbilical hernia defects that are larger than 3 cm. The surgeon must adhere to the principles of tension-free repair to achieve low hernia recurrence rates.

Recommended References and Readings

[1]   Feins, N.R., A. Dzakovic, and K. Papadakis, *Minimally invasive closure of pediatric umbilical hernias. J Pediatr Surg*, 2008. 43(1): p. 127-30.

[2]   Meier, D.E., D.A. OlaOlorun, R.A. Omodele, S.K. Nkor, and J.L. Tarpley, *Incidence of umbilical hernia in African children: redefinition of "normal" and reevaluation of indications for repair. World J Surg*, 2001. 25(5): p. 645-8.

[3]   Muschaweck, U., *Umbilical and epigastric hernia repair. Surg ClinNorth Am*, 2003. 83(5): p. 1207-21.

[4]   Halpern, L.J., *Spontaneous healing of umbilical hernias. JAMA*, 1962. 182: p. 851-2.

[5]   Bevacqua, J., *Umbilical hernias in infants and children. Nurse Pract*, 2009. 34(12): p. 12-3.

[6]   Walker, S.H., *The natural history of umbilical hernia. A six-year follow up of 314 Negro children with this defect. Clin Pediatr* (Phila), 1967. 6(1): p. 29-32.

[7]   Mestel, A.L. and H. Burns, *Incarcerated and strangulated umbilical hernias in infants and children. Clin Pediatr* (Phila), 1963. 2: p. 368-70.

[8] Aslani, N. and C.J. Brown, *Does mesh offer an advantage over tissue in the open repair of umbilical hernias? A systematic review and meta-analysis.* Hernia, 2010. 14(5): p. 455-62.
[9] Mislowsky, A., A. Hemphill, and D.V. Nasrallah, *A scarless technique of umbilical hernia repair in the adult population.* Hernia, 2008. 12(6): p. 627-30.
[10] Halm, J.A., J. Heisterkamp, H.F. Veen, and W.F. Weidema, *Long-term follow-up after umbilical hernia repair: are there risk factors for recurrence after simple and mesh repair.* Hernia, 2005. 9(4): p. 334-7.
[11] Arroyo, A., P. Garcia, F. Perez, J. Andreu, F. Candela, and R. Calpena, *Randomized clinical trial comparing suture and mesh repair of umbilical hernia in adults.* Br J Surg, 2001. 88(10): p. 1321-3.
[12] Venclauskas, L., J. Silanskaite, and M. Kiudelis, *Umbilical hernia: factors indicative of recurrence.* Medicina (Kaunas), 2008. 44(11): p. 855-9.
[13] Kulah, B., I.H. Kulacoglu, M.T. Oruc, A.P. Duzgun, M. Moran, M.M. Ozmen, and F. Coskun, *Presentation and outcome of incarcerated external hernias in adults.* Am J Surg, 2001. 181(2): p. 101-4.
[14] Luijendijk, R.W., M.H. Lemmen, W.C. Hop, and J.C. Wereldsma, *Incisional hernia recurrence following "vest-over-pants" or vertical Mayo repair of primary hernias of the midline.* World J Surg, 1997. 21(1): p. 62-5; discussion 66.
[15] Rodriguez-Hermosa, J.I., A. Codina-Cazador, B. Ruiz-Feliu, J. Roig-Garcia, M. Albiol-Quer, and P. Planellas-Gine, *Incarcerated umbilical hernia in a super-super-obese patient.* Obes Surg, 2008. 18(7): p. 893-5.
[16] Rutkow, I.M., *Demographic and socioeconomic aspects of hernia repair in the United States in 2003.* Surg Clin North Am, 2003. 83(5): p. 1045-51, v-vi.
[17] Andrews, N.J., *Presentation and outcome of strangulated external hernia in a district general hospital.* Br J Surg, 1981. 68(5): p. 329-32.
[18] Martinez-Serrano, M.A., J.A. Pereira, J.J. Sancho, M. Lopez-Cano, E. Bombuy, and J. Hidalgo, *Risk of death after emergency repair of abdominal wall hernias. Still waiting for improvement.* Langenbecks Arch Surg, 2010. 395(5): p. 551-6.
[19] Mayo, W.J., *VI. An Operation for the Radical Cure of Umbilical Hernia.* Ann Surg, 1901. 34(2): p. 276-80.

[20] Roberts, K.E., L. Panait, A.J. Duffy, and R.L. Bell, *Single-port laparoscopic umbilical hernia repair.* Surg Innov, 2010. 17(3): p. 256-60.
[21] Craft, R.O. and K.L. Harold, *Laparoscopic repair of incisional and other complex abdominal wall hernias.* Perm J, 2009. 13(3): p. 38-42.
[22] Hadi, H.I., A. Maw, S. Sarmah, and P. Kumar, *Intraperitoneal tension-free repair of small midline ventral abdominal wall hernias with a Ventralex hernia patch: initial experience in 51 patients.* Hernia, 2006. 10(5): p. 409-13.
[23] Moore, T.C. and H. Siderys, *The use of pliable plastics in the repair of abdominal wall defects.* Ann Surg, 1955. 142(6): p. 973-9.
[24] Kaito, C. and K. Sekimizu, *Colony spreading in Staphylococcus aureus.* J Bacteriol, 2007. 189(6): p. 2553-7.
[25] Bliziotis, I.A., S.K. Kasiakou, A.M. Kapaskelis, and M.E. Falagas, *Mesh-related infection after hernia repair: case report of an emerging type of foreign-body related infection.* Infection, 2006. 34(1): p. 46-8.
[26] Kercher, K.W., R.F. Sing, B.D. Matthews, and B.T. Heniford, *Successful salvage of infected PTFE mesh after ventral hernia repair.* Ostomy Wound Manage, 2002. 48(10): p. 40-2, 44-5.
[27] Paton, B.L., Y.W. Novitsky, M. Zerey, R.F. Sing, K.W. Kercher, and B.T. Heniford, *Management of infections of polytetrafluoroethylene-based mesh.* Surg Infect (Larchmt), 2007. 8(3): p. 337-41.
[28] Petersen, S., G. Henke, M. Freitag, A. Faulhaber, and K. Ludwig, *Deep prosthesis infection in incisional hernia repair: predictive factors and clinical outcome.* Eur J Surg, 2001. 167(6): p. 453-7.
[29] Abramov, D., I. Jeroukhimov, A.M. Yinnon, Y. Abramov, E. Avissar, Z. Jerasy, and O. Lernau, *Antibiotic prophylaxis in umbilical and incisional hernia repair: a prospective randomised study.* Eur J Surg, 1996. 162(12): p. 945-8; discussion 949.
[30] Aufenacker, T.J., M.J. Koelemay, D.J. Gouma, and M.P. Simons, *Systematic review and meta-analysis of the effectiveness of antibiotic prophylaxis in prevention of wound infection after mesh repair of abdominal wall hernia.* Br J Surg, 2006. 93(1): p. 5-10.
[31] Muysoms, F.E., J. Bontinck, and P. Pletinckx, *Complications of mesh devices for intraperitoneal umbilical hernia repair: a word of caution.* Hernia, 2010.
[32] Edelman, D.S. and C.F. Bellows, *Umbilical herniorrhaphy reinforced with biologic mesh.* Am Surg, 2010. 76(11): p. 1205-9.

[33] Ramirez, O.M., E. Ruas, and A.L. Dellon, *"Components separation" method for closure of abdominal-wall defects: an anatomic and clinical study.* Plast Reconstr Surg, 1990. 86(3): p. 519-26.
[34] Hiles, M., R.D. Record Ritchie, and A.M. Altizer, *Are biologic grafts effective for hernia repair?: a systematic review of the literature.* Surg Innov, 2009. 16(1): p. 26-37.
[35] Milburn, M.L., L.H. Holton, T.L. Chung, E.N. Li, G.V. Bochicchio, N.H. Goldberg, and R.P. Silverman, *Acellular dermal matrix compared with synthetic implant material for repair of ventral hernia in the setting of peri-operative Staphylococcus aureus implant contamination: a rabbit model.* Surg Infect (Larchmt), 2008. 9(4): p. 433-42.
[36] Keller, J.E., C.J. Dolce, K.C. Walters, J.J. Heath, R.D. Peindl, K.W. Kercher, A.E. Lincourt, B.T. Heniford, and D.A. Iannitti, *Effect of bacterial exposure on acellular human dermis in a rat ventral hernia model.* J Surg Res, 2010. 162(1): p. 148-52.
[37] Itani, K.M., K. Hur, L.T. Kim, T. Anthony, D.H. Berger, D. Reda, and L. Neumayer, *Comparison of laparoscopic and open repair with mesh for the treatment of ventral incisional hernia: a randomized trial.* Arch Surg, 2010. 145(4): p. 322-8; discussion 328.
[38] Qadri, S.J., M. Khan, S.N. Wani, S.S. Nazir, and A. Rather, *Laparoscopic and open incisional hernia repair using polypropylene mesh - a comparative single centre study.* Int J Surg, 2010. 8(6): p. 479-83.
[39] Sharma, A., M. Mehrotra, R. Khullar, V. Soni, M. Baijal, and P.K. Chowbey, *Laparoscopic ventral/incisional hernia repair: a single centre experience of 1,242 patients over a period of 13 years.* Hernia, 2010.
[40] Carbonell, A.M., K.L. Harold, A.J. Mahmutovic, R. Hassan, B.D. Matthews, K.W. Kercher, R.F. Sing, and B.T. Heniford, *Local injection for the treatment of suture site pain after laparoscopic ventral hernia repair.* Am Surg, 2003. 69(8): p. 688-91; discussion 691-2.
[41] Bencini, L., L.J. Sanchez, M. Bernini, E. Miranda, M. Farsi, B. Boffi, and R. Moretti, *Predictors of recurrence after laparoscopic ventral hernia repair.* Surg Laparosc Endosc Percutan Tech, 2009. 19(2): p. 128-32.
[42] Tse, G.H., B.M. Stutchfield, A.D. Duckworth, A.C. de Beaux, and B. Tulloh, *Pseudo-recurrence following laparoscopic ventral and incisional hernia repair.* Hernia, 2010. 14(6): p. 583-587.

[43] Blatnik, J.A., K.C. Harth, M.I. Aeder, and M.J. Rosen, *Thirty-day readmission after ventral hernia repair: predictable or preventable?* Surg Endosc, 2010.
[44] Bani, D., *Relaxin: a pleiotropic hormone.* Gen Pharmacol, 1997. 28(1): p. 13-22.
[45] Dschietzig, T., C. Bartsch, G. Baumann, and K. Stangl, *Relaxin-a pleiotropic hormone and its emerging role for experimental and clinical therapeutics.* Pharmacol Ther, 2006. 112(1): p. 38-56.
[46] Ghnnam, W.M., A.S. Helal, M. Fawzy, A. Ragab, H. Shalaby, and E. Elrefaay, *Paraumbilical hernia repair during cesarean delivery.* Ann Saudi Med, 2009. 29(2): p. 115-8.
[47] Buch, K.E., P. Tabrizian, and C.M. Divino, *Management of hernias in pregnancy.* J Am Coll Surg, 2008. 207(4): p. 539-42.
[48] Shlomovitz, E., D. Quan, R. Etemad-Rezai, and V.C. McAlister, *Association of recanalization of the left umbilical vein with umbilical hernia in patients with liver disease.* Liver Transpl, 2005. 11(10): p. 1298-9.
[49] McKay, A., E. Dixon, O. Bathe, and F. Sutherland, *Umbilical hernia repair in the presence of cirrhosis and ascites: results of a survey and review of the literature.* Hernia, 2009. 13(5): p. 461-8.
[50] Ammar, S.A., *Management of complicated umbilical hernias in cirrhotic patients using permanent mesh: randomized clinical trial.* Hernia, 2010. 14(1): p. 35-8.
[51] Triantos, C.K., I. Kehagias, V. Nikolopoulou, and A.K. Burroughs, *Surgical Repair of Umbilical Hernias in Cirrhosis With Ascites.* Am J Med Sci, 2010.
[52] Runyon, B.A. and G.L. Juler, *Natural history of repaired umbilical hernias in patients with and without ascites.* Am J Gastroenterol, 1985. 80(1): p. 38-9.
[53] de Goede, B., Jr., H.H. Eker, H.J. Metselaar, H.W. Tilanus, J.F. Lange, and G. Kazemier, *RE: Emergency liver transplantation after umbilical hernia repair: A case report.* Transplant Proc, 2010. 42(7): p. 2823.
[54] Reissfelder, C., B. Radeleff, A. Mehrabi, N.N. Rahbari, J. Weitz, M.W. Buchler, J. Schmidt, and P. Schemmer, *Emergency liver transplantation after umbilical hernia repair: a case report.* Transplant Proc, 2009. 41(10): p. 4428-30.

[55] Leblanc, K.A., *Laparoscopic Hernia Surgery An Operative Guide* 2003, 198 Madison Avenue, New York, NY10016: Oxford University Press Inc. 115-124.

[56] Ji, W., L.T. Li, Z.M. Wang, Z.F. Quan, X.R. Chen, and J.S. Li, *A randomized controlled trial of laparoscopic versus open cholecystectomy in patients with cirrhotic portal hypertension. World J Gastroenterol,* 2005. 11(16): p. 2513-7.

[57] Ozmen, M.M., A. Kessaf Aslar, H.T. Besler, and I. Cinel, *Does splanchnic ischemia occur during laparoscopic cholecystectomy? Surg Endosc,* 2002. 16(3): p. 468-71.

[58] Tuech, J.J., P. Pessaux, N. Regenet, C. Rouge, R. Bergamaschi, and J.P. Arnaud, *Laparoscopic cholecystectomy in cirrhotic patients. Surg Laparosc Endosc Percutan Tech,* 2002. 12(4): p. 227-31.

[59] Thoman, D.S., *Randomized clinical trial comparing suture and mesh repair of umbilical hernia in adults (Br J Surg 2001;88:1321-3). Br J Surg,* 2002. 89(5): p. 627; author reply 628.

[60] Bachman, S. and B. Ramshaw, *Prosthetic material in ventral hernia repair: how do I choose? Surg Clin North Am,* 2008. 88(1): p. 101-12, ix.

[61] Kaafarani, H.M., K. Hur, A. Hirter, L.T. Kim, A. Thomas, D.H. Berger, D. Reda, and K.M. Itani, *Seroma in ventral incisional herniorrhaphy: incidence, predictors and outcome. Am J Surg,* 2009. 198(5): p. 639-44.

[62] Martin, D.F., R.F. Williams, T. Mulrooney, and G.R. Voeller, *Ventralex mesh in umbilical/epigastric hernia repairs: clinical outcomes and complications. Hernia,* 2008. 12(4): p. 379-83.

In: Hernias: Types, Symptoms and Treatment
Editor: James H. Wagner

ISBN: 978-1-61324-125-7
© 2011 Nova Science Publishers, Inc.

Chapter 9

Eventration Disease of the Abdominal Wall

Andrew A. Gassman, Anupama Mehta, Casey Thomas and P. Marco Fisichella[*]

Department of Surgery, Loyola University Medical Center,
Maywood, Illinois, USA

Abstract

Eventration disease is the protrusion of abdominal contents through a defect in the abdominal wall. The hole represents more than an imperfection. It decouples the counterbalancing mechanical forces of the lateral abdominal musculature. This gradual change in abdominal wall mechanics leads to compensatory mechanisms that in turn lead to further herniation. The purpose of this chapter is to comprehensively review the relevant history, pathophysiology, and treatment strategies of ventral incisional hernias.

As there exists a large volume of inconsistent data on methodology of incisional herniorraphy, particular attention has been dedicated to clinical approaches described by evidence-based literature. Additionally, this work includes a detailed discussion of the theory, design, and application of implantable materials. Furthermore, the authors describe the evolution of

---

[*] Corresponding Author: Piero M. Fisichella, MD, Department of Surgery, Loyola University Medical Center, 2160 S First Ave., Maywood, IL 60153, (P) 708-327-2236, (F) 708-327-3492

autologous tissue abdominal wall reconstructive procedures and their evolving integration with minimally invasive technologies. Finally, a brief discussion is held outlining the current evidence that supports mesh fixation techniques.

History of Incisional Hernias

An abdominal wall hernia, also known as ventral hernia, incisional hernia, or eventration, occurs when the abdominal contents push through a weakness in the abdominal wall originating from a previous surgical incision or congenital defect. The balloon-like sac that results may trap a loop of intestine or other abdominal contents, potentially requiring surgery.(1) Joseph-Pierre Desault described the mechanical nature of bowel strangulation present within a hernia in 1798. The risk factors for complication after incisional ventral hernia repair include male sex, age, obesity, jaundice, underlying disease process, wound infection, abdominal distension, pulmonary diseases.(2) Marbury described in 1943 the use of fascial sutures to close incisional hernias. He also reported that it was mechanical forces on the abdominal wall such as obesity, abdominal distention, coughing, and vomiting that predispose a patient to postoperative recurrence. Additional risks include infection and prolonged drainage that weakens or disrupts a wound.(3)

Prior to the 1960's, most incisional hernias were repaired by direct apposition of autogenous tissue. These techniques ran the gamut from simple suture fascial closure to the Nuttall procedure.(4) Nuttall described a repair of the sub-umbilical incisional hernias by "transplantation" of the inferior insertion of the abdominal rectus muscle. It was believed that this approach realigning the muscular fibers in a fashion that re-approximates the ventral fascial layers towards midline and prevented future midline defects. Although there have been modifications, this method did not achieve wide popularity as it is a highly morbid operation.(5) Interestingly, the Nuttall techniques attempted to link the bilateral muscular apparatus of the abdominal wall, a concept that has influenced more recent surgical approaches. (Nuttall FIGURE ###)

The 1960's also saw the growth of synthetic materials' role in eventration disease. Their usage was intermittent until 1959 when Uscher described the use of polypropylene mesh for ventral hernia repair.(6) Over the following decade, the use of mesh and knitted polypropylene synthetic barriers steadily increased.(7) In 1979, Browse and Hurst described a combined approach using flaps of autogenous tissue and synthetic mesh to close large ventral hernia defects. In their report, the rectus abdominis was reflected and subsequently reinforced with polypropylene mesh.(8) Since then many authors have described how to position mesh in relation to the patient's fascia, such as onlay, inlay, underlay, and underlay approaches. In the mid to late 1980's Rives and Stoppa separately described a subfascial, pre-peritoneal approach to the closure of large incisional hernia defects.(9, 10) As we shall discuss later, this approach has become widely adopted.

The advent of a synthetic mesh was not without limitation. The original polypropylene synthetic barriers were relatively stiff. Post-operative patient complaints including rigidity, irritation, pain, and even bowel erosion forced manufacturers to develop lightweight formulations of polypropylene meshes. These newer materials addressed many issues however bowel erosion still represented a catastrophic complication limiting their design. Other products were introduced to address these concerns. For example, expanded polytetraluoroethylene (ePTFE), discovered in the 1930's and used in vascular prosthesis in the 1970's, was first described in the repair ventral hernia defects in 1983.(11) Advanced synthetic material (i.e. ePTFE) usage increased during the 1980's. Concurrently the techniques of laparoscopy and minimally invasive surgery developed advancing the method of mesh insertion and hernia repair. In 1993, LeBlanc and Booth combined both of these technological innovations and described the first laparoscopic incisional hernia repair with ePTFE.(12) Around the same time other innovators took a different approach that revised the use of autogenous tissue to repair large hernia defects. The need to create a lasting repair in a contaminated field prompted the development of these techniques. Specifically, Ramirez, in 1990, described a method to close incisional hernia defects by separating the muscle planes of the abdominal wall termed, component separation.(13) Since then there have been some advancements in the field that have sought to combine both minimally invasive techniques with the insertion of synthetic material and the manipulation of autogenous tissue.

The abdominal wall consists of the rectus abdominis, three layers of lateral musculature, and fascial extension of these muscles. The fascicles of each muscle are directed in different directions to create a strong envelope to contain the abdominal contents.

The rectus muscles act to stabilize both upright posture and the tension exerted by the lateral muscles.

Anatomy of Ventral Incisional Hernia Repair

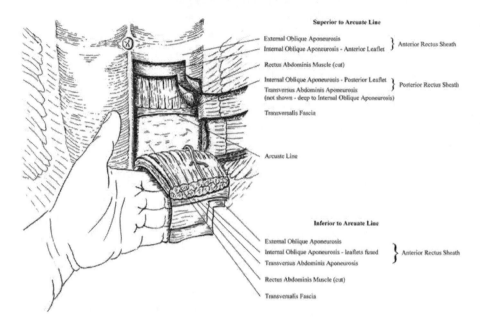

Figure 1. Layers of the abdominal wall. The abdominal wall layers adjacent to the rectus abdominis muscle have been exposed. The rectus sheath above the arcuate line is made of the aponeurosis of external oblique, half of the internal oblique, other half of internal oblique and the transversus abdominal. Below the arcuate line, all 3 aponeuroses pass ventral to rectus muscle. Transversalis fascia makes the dorsal wall of the sheath. The posterior rectus sheath is not a discreet layer below the arcuate line. Lateral to the rectus muscle, the External oblique, Interal oblique and Trans *Copyright Permission:* Practical Plastic Surgery by Zol B Kryger and Mark Sisco, Landes Bioscience published in Austin, Texas in 2007. Page 265.

The linea alba is the area between the rectus muscles where each side's muscular aponeurosis extends beyond the rectus and meets in the anterior midline. The triple crossing pattern provides the strength to the midline aponeurosis. Although this area is named as a line, it more often represents an area than a "line", particular in the setting of herniation. During respiration and coughing in the setting of eventration, the abdominal muscles including fibers of the *linea alba* exert lateral distracting forces which result in increased fascial tension making the defect larger.(14) As such, the hernia is more than a hole in the abdominal wall. It is a mechanical weakening that decouples the bilateral muscular apparatus that contributes to breathing, body positioning, and truncal movements.

The mechanical characteristics associated with ventral midlines hernias different than other types of hernia (i.e. inguinal, obturator, etc). The mechanical decoupling of the ventral midline defects can contribute to respiratory insufficiency. To compensate the affected individual will expend more effort on the accessory respiratory muscles. While doing so, abdominal wall movement in and out during both inspiration and expiration is exaggerated. Bowels are pushed out on inspiration and eventually the bowels lose their right of domain. As the back muscles are not counterbalanced by abdomen an individual may experience gradual postural changes occur (i.e. lordosis). Over time the lateral abdominal muscles retract and become increasingly fatty and fibrotic. Thus, the lateral muscular retraction both makes defect larger and harder to repair as the muscular physiology of the abdominal wall changes.

Dubay et al., developed a rat model to describe the pathological changes that occur when lateral muscular retracts in response to ventral incisional hernia. They specifically harvested internal oblique muscle fiber from rats that had either surgically created hernias or sham operation.(15) These fibers were analyzed for length density and collagen content. They found that the hernia group had shorter, fibrotic, and atrophied fibers. This data suggests that once ventral anatomy is lost, there is an increased load to midline resulting in difficult fascial re-approximation. Subsequently, an incisional hernia can set off a cyclic self-perpetuating process for recurrence when proper anatomic configuration is not recreated by appropriate repair.

Hernia Biology

Type 1 collagen has the highest tensile strength of all collagen filaments and is predominantly found in bone, fascia, and skin. The quantity and quality of type 1 collagen is important for hernia formation and recurrence. For example, individuals with inherent defects in collagen production such as Ehlers-Danlos syndrome, Marfan's syndrome, and osteogenesis imperfecta syndrome, have increased incidence of hernia formation and recurrence. Klinge et al., examined the wounds of individuals with recurrent hernias. They found by western blot analysis that tissue along the hernia repair in this population demonstrates both decreased levels of the type 1 collagen and metalloproteinases, the proteins responsible for collagen protein remodeling.(16)

Growth factors are in flux in the wound bed after incisional hernia repair. DiVita et al. documented that the fluid present in the wounds of primary incisional hernia repairs is initially high in concentration of growth factors such as Fibroblast Growth Factor (FGF) and these values fall significantly on postoperative day one.(17) Growth factors such as FGF recruit of inflammatory cells that produce collagen and other connective tissue substrates. Dubay et al. examined if there was a means to biologically alter the rate of hernia formation by influencing collagen deposition by prolonged administration of growth factor in a rat ventral incisional hernia wound model. They found that bFGF, administered as a slow-release depot from a polydioxanone (PDS) substrate, significantly increased the tensile strength of a wound and subsequently decreased the rate of hernia formation by 63%. Immunohistochemical analysis of the treatment group demonstrated both increased angiogenesis and collagen protein production.(15) Other pro-angiogenic growth factors have also demonstrated similar results (i.e. TGF-ß).(18)

Clinical Observations

Primary vs. Mesh-Based Repairs

During the first 30 postoperative days the tensile strength of a wound is at it weakest. The majority of the repair's integrity relies primarily on the strength of the implanted material and repair technique. The implanted material and repair technique also play a major role in a repair's longevity. As recurrence rate is perhaps one the most important and widely studies features related to incisional hernia repair, the repair method and material fall under high degrees of scrutiny. For example, both Sahlin and Roberts studied the recurrence rates associated with primary repair. They found that there was no difference in recurrence rate for primary repairs performed with either monofilament or braided suture. Additionally, there was no difference for repairs performed in a running or interrupted fashion. (19, 20) As we shall see, each element in the repair of a ventral incisional hernia has been closely evaluated.

Since its wide usage began in the 1950's, synthetic mesh has been compared in relation to primary suture repair of ventral incisional hernia. However no controlled trials were performed to evaluate this fact specifically until relatively recently. Luijendijk et al., found that at 3-years, regardless of hernia size, mesh repair was statistically superior to suture repair (43% vs. 24%) in the recurrence of midline abdominal incisional hernias.(21) Follow-up work by Burger documented a 10-year cumulative recurrence rate of 63% for suture repair and 32% for underlay mesh repairs of first time midline incisional hernia defects <6cm. (22)

Tension is a feature common to both primary and mesh repairs that is critical to successful repair. More specifically, multiple authors abdicate that excessive tension at the time of wound closure is a significant contributor to repair failure, local swelling, and wound separation.(21) As such, "tension-free" repairs have been the main thrust of mesh based repairs. To accomplish this goal there appears to be a general agreement that the overlap of mesh with autogenous abdominal tissue needs to be at the very least 3 cm. This allows a suitable surface area for connective tissue growth as well as fixation of the prosthesis within the abdominal wall. The wide placement allows for the shrinkage of the mesh, secondarily to fibrovascular invasion, and decreases the risk of recurrent hernia occurring at the lateral edge of the defect.(23)

Mesh Placement in Relation to Fascia

The surgeon must know where to place a mesh when planning to repair an incisional hernia. Hawn et al., performed a retrospective review of 1,346 incisional hernia repairs using Cox regression models. They found that the effectiveness of mesh repair varied by its position. Specifically, when compared to suture repair, open underlay mesh repair (hazard ratio = 0.72) and laparoscopic intraperitoneal repair (hazard ratio = 0.49) significantly reduced the risk of recurrence. However mesh onlay or inlay had no improvement over primary suture repair.(24)

Rives and Stoppa independently described a method of repairing ventral hernias.(9, 10) Their method has become widely accepted as a standard for open incisional hernia repair. The basis of this repair is a large overlap of underlay mesh that allows for distribution of forces over the entire mesh thus decreasing the pressure at the defect itself, leading to reduced recurrence. In brief, the mesh is placed deep to the rectus abdominis muscles and superficial to the posterior fascia. The peritoneum and/or posterior fascia is closed deep to the mesh to protect the underlying bowel from the foreign material. The mesh is secured circumferentially with "U" stitch sutures placed full thickness through the abdominal wall and mesh and brought out through separate skin incisions.

However there are significant considerations that come with this procedure. The open approach requires extensive soft tissue dissection of already compromised tissue, and the operating surgeon must protect against skin flap necrosis, seroma formation, and local infection.

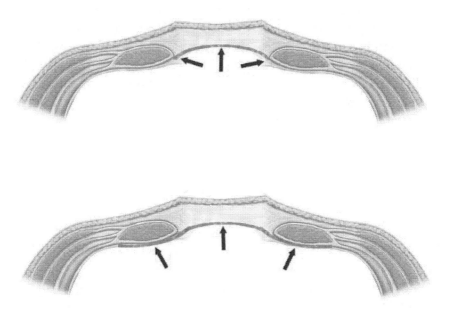

Figure 2. Pressure and Overlap: Retraction of lateral muscle groups and increases of intra-abdominal pressure both compromise the integrity of inlay mesh repairs. A large overlap of underlying mesh is important to allow for distribution of forces over entire mesh. This decreases pressure at the defect itself an helps ensure apposition of mesh and fascia along the periphery.

When Rives and Stoppa described their pre-peritoneal reconstruction method only synthetic meshes with a high tendency to erode intra-abdominal organs were available. Without more inert prosthetic materials, peritoneal coverage and omental flaps were necessary. Since then several composite synthetic materials have been develop specifically to prevent visceral injury and adhesion formation. Wiliams et al., demonstrated that the Rives-Stoppa method, could be accomplished intra-peritoneally. Specifically, they performed open incisional hernia repairs using an intraperitoneal mesh underlay. In their study, the repairs were completed with a variety materials designed to limit visceral erosion including ePTFE, coated polyester, coated polypropylene, and biologic meshes. With mean 1-year follow up, the overall recurrence rate was 3.4%. Their overall complication rate was 26%, with seroma formation being the most frequent at 16%.(25) Gullion et al., also examined the effect intraperitoneal placement of ePTFE mesh has on recurrence and complication rates for ventral incisional hernias. The 3-year follow up of 158 patients revealed only 4% serious postoperative complications (i.e. sepsis requiring mesh removal). Although there were minor inconsistencies between the analysis groups there were comparable long-term complications and recurrences for both extraperitoneal and intraperitoneal incisional hernia mesh repairs (3% and 4%). (26) Overall, these studies demonstrate that with an appropriate material intraperitoneal mesh repair is similar to extraperitoneal placement in both safety and recurrence rate.

Laparoscopic vs. Open Repairs

Laparoscopy has proven to be a valuable tool in the treatment of eventration disease since LeBlanc and Booth first described laparoscopic ventral incisional hernia repair in 1993. Over a mean 42 month follow-up, laparoscopic repairs have been described to have a recurrence rate of 2.9% and 10% morbidity (i.e. seroma, pain, surgical site infection and recurrence combined).(27) Many authors have compared laparoscopic and open ventral hernia repairs to specifically see if one technique is superior to another. In fact, the myriad of studies vary by design, materials, techniques, retrospective or prospective design.(28-30) To gain some clarity, several authors independently performed meta-analyses to draw conclusions from a potentially larger cohort. Although we must grant that such methods do not correct each studies fundamental errors and the data analysis has to be carefully inspected for inconsistencies, these data sets do allow authors to gain greater understanding of the population as whole.

Recurrence

Pierce et al., performed a meta-analysis of studies that dealt with either laparoscopic ventral hernia repair alone or performed in comparison with an open repair. Their pooled analysis included 45 published series over a ten-year period (1996-2006). . Seventy-three percent of these studies were retrospective and included a total of 5340 patients. Of these individuals, 1377 patients were from series that directly compared laparoscopic with open repairs. During that time period recurrence rates for the paired studies were 12% for open and 4% for laparoscopic repairs. Although both open and laproscopic patients had similar demographic and operative characteristics, the laparoscopic repair group typically had bigger hernia defects (by 17.1 sq cm), subsequently requiring larger pieces of mesh (by 90.8 sq cm). The average follow-up period for these studies was 20 months for open repairs and 17 months for laparoscopic repairs.(31)

Over a longer period of follow up the recurrence rates for laparoscopic repairs appear to approach levels comparable to open repair. Cheng et al. performed a decision tree analysis of 33 studies that included precise herniation rates after both open and laparoscopic abdominal surgery. The pooled 3-year incidence from these studies found the annual incidence rate 6.6% 2.2% 0.7% for post-operative years 1, 2, and 3 respectively. There was a cumulative incidence of 9.5% in these 11,364 surgeries at 3 years.(32) These results are much better in terms of recurrence than the primary repair however this recurrence rate is at least as much as rates quoted elsewhere with the open Rives-Stoppa method.(25, 26) Similarly, Forbes et al. also performed a meta-analysis of randomized control trials comparing laparoscopic and open closure of ventral incisional hernia defects. Their analysis included 8 studies for a total of 517 patients. Their analysis revealed that there was no significant difference between groups in hernia recurrence rates.(33)

On a side note, Cheng also examined a problem specific to the laparoscopic approach, the port site hernia. As this complication is unique to the Laparoscopic repair, it is important to understand prior to completing a benefit/risk analysis comparison between open and laparoscopic incisional hernia repair. They found that for 3,880 laparoscopic procedures over the same 3-year time frame the cumulative incidence of port site hernia was 0.69%.(32)

Complications and Length of Stay

Several studies have examined what benefits, besides recurrence rates, laparoscopy offers over the open repair of ventral incisional hernias. For example Rudmik et al. reviewed 8 studies, including a total of 712 patients, which directly compared open and laparoscopic approaches. They found that individuals who underwent a laparoscopic repair were 58% less likely to develop a post-operative complication and on average required half as many hospital days as their open counterparts (2 vs. 4 days). (34) Forbes et al. demonstrated work that echoed these results. Their meta-analysis of randomized control trials comparing laparoscopic and open closure of ventral incisional hernia defects. Their analysis included 8 studies for a total of 517 patients. Although the duration of surgery varied amongst the studies evaluated, the mean length of hospital stay was shorter after laparoscopic repair in six of their included studies. Specifically, the longest mean stay was 5-7 days for laparoscopic and 10 days for open surgery. Laparoscopic hernia repair was associated with fewer bleeding complications, wound infections, and infections requiring mesh removal.(33) Additionally, a meta-analysis performed by Goodney et al., also found that perioperative complications (14% vs. 27%) and average length of stay were approximately half for the laparoscopic groups.(35) Pierce's meta-analysis directly comparing 1377 patients who underwent laparoscopic or open repairs demonstrated a total wound complication rate of 16.8% for open repairs and 5.3% for laparoscopic repairs. Infections were document in 10.4% of open repairs and 2.3% of laparoscopic repairs. Of note, seroma formation was equal for both repair types (12%). The average length of hospital stay for laparoscopic repair was half that of an open repair (2 vs. 4 days).(31)

Quality of Life

Hope et al. examined what role laparoscopic surgery played on a patient's quality of life during the first 6 months post-operatively. In 56 patients, who had no significant difference in pre-operative assessment of quality of life, those patient who underwent a laparoscopic repair overall had a statistically significant improvement in their perception of general health, vitality, and mental health. Additionally laproscopically treated patients also noted improved comfort and ability to rejoin activities such as walking and general exercise.(36)

Although large data sets can present some challenges in congruence between studies, they do provide a broader picture of how a particular treatment strategy has performed over a larger population subset. These large studies indicate that laparoscopic repair of ventral incisional hernia are at least similar to an open Rives-Stoppa ventral incisional repair in recurrence rate. Depending on the data in question, one may argue that it may in fact be better. A laparoscopic repair is, however, consistently superior to an open repair in terms of its reduced complication rate, decreased post-operative hospital length of stay, and increased patient satisfaction.

Incarceration and Contamination

The incarcerated ventral hernia presents a unique set of challenges to the operating surgeon. These hernias require expedient repair to avoid bowel necrosis, surgical site contamination, and sepsis. The use of polypropylene has been described in the contaminated surgical wound.(37) However surgical contamination is widely regarded as a contraindication to prosthetic insertion. For example, surgical site infections have been described to occur 32% of the clean contaminated wounds and 36% of the contaminated wounds in open repairs. Of those infections, 57% of the clean contaminated wounds and 50% of the contaminated wounds required some surgical intervention such as debridement, washout, or removal. (38) These rates generally deter most surgeons from inserting prosthetic material in a contaminated field. Additionally, instances of contamination or bowel compromise, such as incarceration or enterotomy, are considered contraindication to laparoscopic repair. For example, Franklin et al., reviewed 240 incisional ventral hernias. In their work, 96% of individuals were repaired laproscopically and 4% were done open due to dense adhesion formation and bowel involvement. The majority of cases involved polypropylene mesh, however if a contaminated field was present biologic mesh or primary laparoscopic repair was performed.(27) Their results reflect that common belief common to ventral incisional hernia repair.

Some authors challenge the notion that bowel involvement and contamination are contra-indications to both laparoscopic and mesh repairs. For example, Shah et al. abdicated that at least bowel incarceration is not a contra-indication to a laparoscopic repair. They treated 112 patients with incarcerated primary ventral and incisional hernias via laparoscopic repair. In their series, 103 patients were able to be successfully treated laproscopically with mesh repair. This group included individuals with either an enterotomy (4%) or non-viable bowel requiring laparoscopic resection. In their retrospective review they found that a laparoscopic approach is a safe means to repair these ventral defects with < 3 % recurrence rates and only 1 patient in their cohort requiring mesh removal due to infection. (39) Diaz et al., also found that biologic meshes are useful in the treatment of ventral hernias in the presence of a contaminated field. Specifically, their case series used acellular human dermis to repair 75 hernias that were in either clean contaminated or contaminated/dirty wounds.(40) They found that 33% of these wounds subsequently developed an infection and just over half of that subgroup required subsequent removal. The specific difference between mesh materials will be described at greater length below.

Mesh Material

Mesh is the reinforcing substrate that augments native tissue structural characteristics during hernia repair. Each unique mesh design has its own particular advantages and specific complication risks. Ideally a mesh is chemically inert so as to limit local inflammation, hypersensitivity reaction, and carcinogenesis. The material must have physical integrity to withstand the manipulation of insertion and the mechanical forces present along the abdominal wall. Additionally the material should have compliance characteristics that match the abdominal wall. If the mesh is placed intrabdominally, then it should allow adequate tissue ingrowth to foster integration yet prevent the formation adhesion and sinus tract formation to visceral organs. The material should have the ability to be sterilized preoperatively and a resistance to infection after insertion. It is also important that the mesh causes no change in abdominal wall compliance that would alter the function of muscles responsible for movement and breathing.(41) Finally all these features should be accomplished at a price point that makes the device accessible.

Currently available meshes can be grossly divided into synthetic and biologic varieties. Synthetic meshes are typically comprised of polypropylene (PP), polyester (PE), and ePTFE. Although they have great strength characteristics, PP and PE meshes alone are typically not used in abdominal procedures as they foster dense visceral adhesion formation with risk of fistula tract formation. Instead, these materials when used join another barrier material creating a composite mesh. These barrier materials are usually degradable biologic substrates such as collagen derivatives, polyethylene glycol, polydioxanone, glycerol, or hyaluronic acid derivatives. Biologic meshes and ePTFE, due to different biochemical and porosity characteristics, do not generate as dense adhesion formation. Thus, they do not require additionally layers for visceral protection. Chelala et al., evaluated the rate of adhesion formation of composite mesh over an 8-year period. They retrospectively reviewed the records of 733 individuals who underwent a laparoscopic incisional ventral hernia repair with Parietex™ composite mesh. Eighty-five individuals required additional laparoscopy for a myriad of reasons including recurrence, elective gastrointestinal surgery, and emergent surgery. They found that all meshes had a neo-peritoneum and 89% of individuals had minor to no adhesions against the prosthesis.(42)

The porosity of a mesh determines how much it will interact with surrounding tissue. To promote native tissue ingrowth fenestrations or interstices are created and manipulated with in the material. Pores increase the effective area that mesh is in contact with recipient tissue. Large holes allow tissue, rich in both inflammatory cells and fibroblasts, to grow through and envelop the mesh itself. Porosity does not confer specificity to a specific type of tissue in-growth. As such, meshes with large pores risk the formation of adhesion or sinus tract to visceral organs. However, composite meshes are typically designed with large pore materials placed against the abdominal wall to allow integration and small pore or nonporous material placed towards abdominal contents to prevent these complications. No large prospective studies have been performed analyzing the role porosity plays on subsequent intra-abdominal adhesion formation.

After insertion of exogenous material there are a few key steps that must happen before a material is integrated. Local inflammatory cascades bring both neutraphils and macrophages. These cells then recruit fibroblasts and endothelial cells, which in turn form collagen tissue substrates and neovascularization, respectively. The degree to which the implanted substrate stimulates this initial inflammatory reaction and is subsequent remodeling is determined by the material's biocompatibility characteristics. A full discussion of specific synthetic materials degradation characteristics is beyond the focus of this review. However, the reader should understand that current nonabsorbable, implantable mesh will undergo the majority of it fibrovascular ingrowth within the first 2 weeks post-implantation.

Biologic meshes are synthetic sheets of biopolymers, such as collagen and elastin, derived from human or animal extracellular matrices. Theses meshes, procured from a variety of tissue donors that range from pericardium, dermis, and intestinal submucosa are decellularized to limit antigenicity. The remaining tissue serves as a substrate for host tissue and capillary ingrowth from the surrounding wound bed. They develop their neovascular in-growth secondarily to collagenases and metalloproteases. The degree of early parenchymal invasion and integration far exceeds levels found in synthetics like ePTFE.(43) Silverman demonstrated in a porcine model that acellular dermis, such as Alloderm, has superior long-term integration compared to ePTFE at 9 months.(44) Although the cellular recruitment also leads to significant contracture, the integrated tissue demonstrated robust capillary networks.(43) These neovasculatures potentially allow the recipient to recruit host immune function to the surgical site. As such these products boast the ability to clear modest infection adjacent to the implanted material.

Positioning of a biologic mesh is key to its success. Espinosa-de-los-Monteros et al. analyzed the role biologic meshes such as acellular human dermis plays in open hernia repair. They found that compared to case matched controls that underwent primary closure, the addition of human cadaveric acellular dermis as an overlay to that repair resulted in a significant decrease in recurrence rate. They postulated that this was secondary to an added layer of strength in the repair. Of note, there was no difference in operative morbidity with addition this biologic mesh. Local complications were fewer (26% vs. 33%) but these findings were not statistically significant.(45)However, Candage et al. found that when a biologic mesh is used as an inlay bridging fascial edges that recurrence rates approached 80%.(46) Recurrent eventration was also noted secondary to eventual laxity of the dermal substrate.

Several biologic mesh manufacturers manipulate their product to limit the substrates degradation over time. Manufacturer based studies, such as the work by Sandor et al., demonstrated that steps inherent in biologic mesh fabrication such as chemical crosslinking are vitally important to cellular invasion, fibroblast recruitment, integration, contracture, and eventual graft laxity. (47) Furthermore, several authors have documented that chemical crosslinking limits both enzymatic degradation and the tissue penetration by mesh recipients cell. (48, 49) It would seem that cross-linked biologic meshes gain the ability to limit degradation at the expense of one of the substrates greatest advantages in contaminated fields, the ability to recruit and integrate with recipient's immune system.

Biologic meshes have demonstrated great promise. However no clear consensus is currently present. Although some authors have described the use of biologic meshes as adjunct in laparoscopic surgery, no trials have been performed comparing its use between open and laparoscopic approaches. Furthermore, biologic meshes are relatively new alternatives for abdominal wall reconstruction there have been few randomized trials comparing these substrates head to head, and those studies are limited by small sample size, lack of proper controls, and short follow up. (50, 51)

Component Separation Repairs

The component separation technique for abdominal wall reconstruction, originally described by Ramirez et al.(13), involves separating the muscles of the abdominal wall and transposing their position to closure a hernia defect.

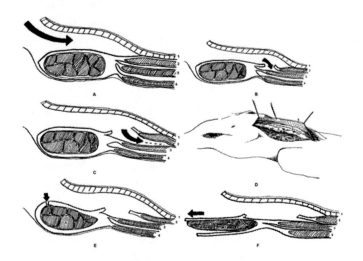

Figure 3. Component Separation: Originally described by Ramirez and colleagues. After entering the abdominal cavity, the bowels are dissected free from the ventral abdominal wall. (1A) The skin and subcutaneous fat (1) are dissected free from the anterior sheath of the rectus abdominal muscle (5) and the aponeurosis of the external oblique muscle (2). (1B and 1C) The aponeurosis of the external oblique muscle (2) is transected longitudinally about 2 cm lateral from the rectus sheath, including the muscular part on the thoracic wall, which extends at least 5 to 7 cm cranially of the costal margin. (1D) The external oblique muscle (2) is separated from the internal oblique muscle (3), as far laterally as possible. (1E and 1F) If primary closure is impossible with undue tension, a further gain of 2 to 4 cm can be reached by separation of the posterior rectal sheath from the rectus abdominal muscle (5). Care must be taken not to damage the blood supply and the nerves that run between the internal oblique and transverse (4) muscle and enter the rectus abdominal muscle at the posterior side. *Copyright permission*: de Vries Reilingh T, et al. "'Components Separation Technique' for the Repair of Large Abdominal Wall Hernias. *J Am Coll Surg*. Vol. 196, No. 1, January 2003.

More specifically, after the elevation of extensive lateral skin flaps the external oblique muscle is detached from its medial insertion on the rectus sheath along the entire semi-lunar line. The external oblique muscle is subsequently elevated off of the internal oblique muscle. The horizontal translation of the musculature allows for greater approximation of the midline fascial elements. Additionally, separation of the posterior rectus sheath from the rectus muscle itself may be performed for additional intra-abdominal domain recovery. (FIGURE: #3)

The component separation technique has been well described as an alternate repair in contaminated fields when implantation of synthetic mesh material is a concern.(52) De Vries Reilingh et al., described the use of this technique for complex ventral hernia repair in both clean and contaminated surgical fields. Over a 1 to 4 year follow-up period, their work documented a recurrence rate that ranged from 4-30%. Additionally, wound complication (i.e. seroma, surgical site infection, etc.) rates varied from 1-84%. This variation was owed in part to variation in technique between the studies described. The higher wound complications were owed in part to the subsequent vascular compromise to the overlying skin flaps inherent the extensive surgical dissection.(53).

Vascular compromise appeared to the main limitation to Ramirez's component separation. Several authors worked independently to solve this problem. Maas et al. described a modification to the technique that avoided flap ischemia. In their method, myofascial separation is accomplished by carrying the dissection directly down over the medial insertion of the external oblique. This modification saves the patient from significant skin flap elevation. (54) Around this time, Lowe et al. described a case series where they performed component separation by endoscopically dissecting the tissue free in a plane just superficial to the external oblique.(55) Their data reflected similar recurrence rates but decrease wound complications when compared to the conventional open component separation. Maas' group then described an endoscopic variation of their modified technique. Specifically they dissected a plane between the external and internal oblique muscles, originating at the aponeurosis of the external oblique, using a combination of open and video-assisted balloon dissection. Once they developed an inter-muscular plane, the aponeurosis was divided from within the potential space under video guidance. They report no wound complications (i.e. hematoma, seroma, or local infection) in their small series with variable follow-up (i.e. 2-24 months). (56)

Limited wound complications have made laparoscopy and minimally invasive techniques particularly enticing to surgeons who perform and study the component separation. Rosen et al. examined the potential difference in the degree of fascial advancement open and laproscopically assisted component separation procedures. (57)In a porcine model, they found that the laparoscopic component separation resulted yielded 86% of the fascial advancement they could obtain with an open procedure, regardless of procedural contamination. Specifically, their demonstrated case series entailed individuals with multiple comorbidities (i.e. smokers, BMI >35, etc) that required removal of infected abdominal wall prostheses. In this small series, there was a mid-line wound that did not affect the lateral ports, but no hernia recurred in the 5-month follow up.(58)

Component separation gains additional benefit with the addition of mesh. Ko et al. examined the role mesh augmentation plays in the complex ventral hernia repair. In their retrospective review 200 patients underwent component separation. Two groups of 18 patients had either a biologic, conventional polypropylene, or lightweight polypropylene meshes placed as an underlay. Over a mean follow-up of 10 months, they found that the component separation alone had a recurrence rate of 23% while the biologic, conventional polypropylene, or lightweight polypropylene mesh groups had mean recurrence rates of 33%, 16% and 0% respectively. (59) It is also important to note that lightweight polypropylene was not used during concomitant bowel surgery or in contaminated fields. Bachman et al. later found similar results.(60)

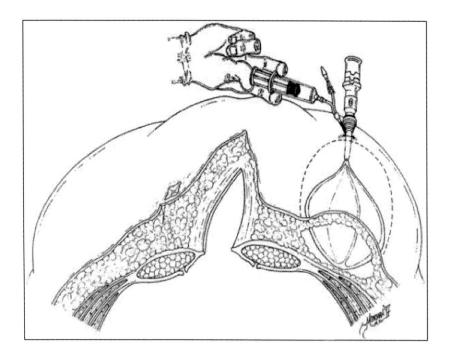

Figure 4a and 4b. (Continued).

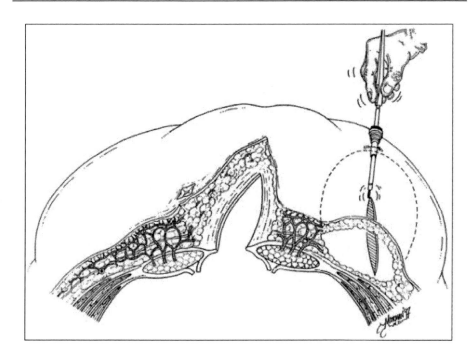

Figure 4a and 4b. Endoscopically assisted component separation: Endoscopic dissection of the tissue plane superficial to external oblique. A plane of dissection is created between external and internal oblique. Open and video-assisted balloon dissection is used to create inter-muscular plane. *Copyright permission*: Lowe J et al: "Endoscopically assisted 'Components Separation' for closure of abdominal wall defects., *Plastic and Reconstructive Surgery.* 105 (2): 720 – 730, February 2000.

Malik et al., presented a small case series that combined elements of standard laparoscopic ventral hernia repair with laparoscopic assisted component separation. Their worked once again described balloon dissection between the external and internal oblique muscles and subsequent laparoscopic division. In their hands this allowed 6-8 cm. of fascial tissue release on each side. Trocar ports, through the same, skin incisions were advanced into the abdominal cavity. Malik then described approximation of the rectus by intracorporeal suturing the medial aspect of each rectus sheath with PFTE suture. Finally, they completed their repair by tacking a composite mesh under their medialized rectus muscles with 5cm of overlap and fixing in place with both tacks and trans-fascial sutures. At a little over 3 months post op, there were no recurrences or wound complications. Although these results represent a small series with short follow – up, the results are promising for this multi-modality repair.(61)

Staged Repair

Patients that have significant loss of domain require additional considerations for their reconstruction. Tran et al. performed a retrospective review of bilateral staged abdominal wall reconstruction using tissue expanders for significant abdominal wall defects with considerable loss of domain. They used tissue expanders in either the subcutaneous or intermuscular planes (between the external and internal oblique muscles). In their series, the average hernia defect area was 333 sq cm for subcutaneous tissue expansion and 1,134 sq cm for intermuscular placement. After these prosthesis underwent gradual dilation on an outpatient basis (average 90 days), the patient returned to the operating room for completion of their separation of components procedure. Twenty-nine percent of cases from either strategy required subsequent reinforcement with a synthetic mesh. Overall there were lower recurrence rates in the intermuscular expansion group (i.e. 26% vs. 33% over an average 3-4 year follow up period). These results demonstrate that access and dilation of the intermuscular plane is superior to separation of components procedures in patients with a large loss of domain.

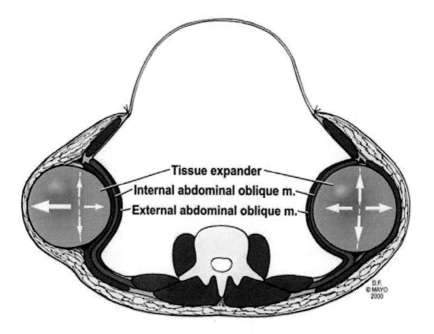

Figure 5. (Continued).

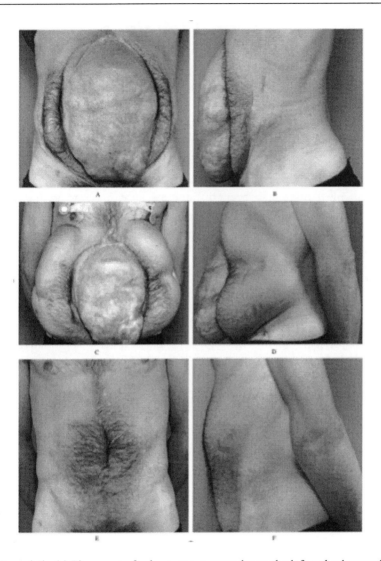

Figure 5a and 5b. (a) Placement of subcutaneous expander on the left and submuscular expander on the right beneath external oblique muscle. Benefit in those patients with loss of domain. (b) Forty-two-year-old man with necrotizing pancreatitis underwent 15 debridements, vicryl mesh closure, and a split thickness skin graft. Submuscular expander placement allowed successful closure of hernia without synthetic mesh. He was without recurrent hernia after 5 years. *Copyright permission*: Tran N et al: "Tissue Expansion-Assisted Closure of Massive Ventral Hernias". *J Am Coll Surg*. 196 (3): 484 – 488, March 2003.

Fixation Technique

Mesh has the advantage of providing hernia repairs with additional support. However fixing that mesh into position presents the operating surgeon with additional considerations. Much like the mesh itself, the addition of fixation material exposes patients to the same risks of foreign body insertion (i.e. local inflammation, nidus for infection, erosion in adjacent structures, etc). During open repairs mesh are typically fixed with suture and during laparoscopic repairs they are held in place using either tacks or transfascial sutures. Comparison of these means of fixation has been difficult because once again there are no randomized control trial that match fixation technique while controlling for patient risk factors, operative technique and material.

Witkowski et al. studied the frank need for fixation in open repairs. They found that tacks or transfascial sutures are not necessary for successful open, preperitoneal ventral incisional hernias repair with polypropylene mesh. They dissected free the preperitoneal space and re-approximated the posterior rectus sheath. As pain is a common complaint associate with large mesh, Rives-Stoppa ventral hernia repair, Witkowski and colleagues upheld that removing mesh fixation by creating a submuscular or preperitoneal pocket alleviates some of that post-operative pain. Additionally they noted that inconsistent fixation leads to mesh folding and the development of a potential space around the mesh resulting in seroma formation.(62)

Laproscopic repairs cannot rely on preperitoneal pockets. As such, a myriad of highly debated options exist for mesh fixation during laparoscopic repairs. This question was initially addressed in an animal model. Melman et al. compared various laparoscopic fixation techniques on biologic mesh to porcine peritoneal surface. They directly compared the acute fixation strength of 0-prolene suture, absorbable tacks, non-absorbable tacks, and various fibrin sealant products. They found that the acute fixation strength was greatest for suture, followed by non absorbable tacks, then absorbable tacks, and least for fibrin sealant.(63) However, Eriksen et al. examined fixation at longer time points and found in their porcine hernia model that there was no difference in the type of fixation (titanium tacks or fibrin glue) at 30 day. Although there was some mesh folding during the study that could be associated with future hernia formation, no actual hernia recurrences were found at 1 month in this porcine model.(64) Of note, some anatomical considerations must be taken into account when drawing comparisons between porcine and human hernia repair as each species carries their weight and intra-abdominal contents differently.

Clinical trials have shown that the exact type of intra-abdominal fixation technique is not critical to recurrence. Perrone et al. performed a prospective trial comparing laparoscopic hernia repair techniques for 116 patients over a median of 22 months. They had an overall complication rate of 27% and recurrence rate of 9.3%. Sixty-five percent of repairs were performed with transfascial sutures and the remainder was performed with only tack fixation. They found similar recurrence rates for the transfascial suture group and the tack-alone group, 9.2 and 8.5%, respectively.(65) Additionally, Rudmik et al. performed an extensive literature review analyzing many features associated with laparoscopic ventral hernia repair, including fixation technique. In their search, they found 7 studies that utilized tack fixation alone (1,156 patients) and 13 studies employed transfacial sutures for intraperitoneal fixation (2,234). Their review found similar recurrence rates for both types of repair (4.5 and 4.4% respectively).(34)

Conclusion

The treatment of eventration disease is a complex endeavor that requires more than just patching a hole. Formal reconstruction that reconnects the bilateral muscular apparatus has the potential cure to the disease. However, as the operative dissection required can be quite extensive, the surgeon must judiciously choose the level of repair suitable for the patient given their comorbidities, extent of herniation, and overall risk of recurrence. Fortunately for the surgeon a myriad of new surgical techniques and materials are available to improve the longevity of an abdominal wall repair under even the most contaminated situations. These technologies also represent a challenge to the surgeon as they must stay abreast of these treatment modalities to truly provide their patients with the greatest number of options and most individual treatment plans.

A surgeon must have a general set of goals in mind when setting out to reconstruct the ventral abdominal wall. These principles should carry over through a variety of approaches and clinical scenarios so as to allow the surgeon to perform successful repairs in a variety of clinical settings when tools or materials can vary from institution. Firstly, the procedure must be both safe and effective. As a physician we must ensure that we first do no harm to our patient and minimize the possible untoward risks carried by any surgical procedure. The surgeon must strive to perform procedures that will result in low recurrence rates. Additionally, a surgeon should be limit the rate by which a patient develops complications (i.e. hematoma, seroma, wound infection, etc.). While private industry continues to develop myriad of solutions to meet these needs, it is the surgeon that must decipher what products represent advancements of the science. To this end, additional randomized control trials are required to generate quality evidence that demonstrates what elements of incisional hernia repair are truly necessary.

References

[1] Pham CT, Perera CL, Watkin DS, Maddern GJ. Laparoscopic ventral hernia repair: a systematic review. *Surg Endosc.* 2009 Jan;23(1):4-15.

[2] Millikan KW. Incisional hernia repair. *Surg Clin North Am.* 2003 Oct;83(5):1223-34.

[3] Marbury WB. Postoperative hernia: Report of a case of repair with fascial sutures. *The American Journal of Surgery.* 1943;59(1):60-7.

[4] Nuttall HC. Rectus Transplantation in the Treatment of Ventral Herniae. *Br Med J.* 1926 Jan 23;1(3395):138-9.

[5] Tentes AA, Xanthoulis AI, Mirelis CG, Bougioukas IG, Tsalkidou EG, Bekiaridou KA, et al. Nuttall technique: A method for subumbilical incisional hernia repair revised. *Langenbecks Arch Surg.* 2008 Mar;393 (2):191-4.

[6] Usher FC, Fries JG, Ochsner JL, Tuttle LL, Jr. Marlex mesh, a new plastic mesh for replacing tissue defects. II. Clinical studies. *AMA Arch Surg.* 1959 Jan;78(1):138-45.

[7] Jacobs E, Blaisdell FW, Hall AD. Use of knitted marlex mesh in the repair of ventral hernias. *Am J Surg.* 1965 Dec;110(6):897-902.

[8] Browse NL, Hurst P. Repair of long, large midline incisional hernias using reflected flaps of anterior rectus sheath reinforced with Marlex mesh. *Am J Surg.* 1979 Nov;138(5):738-9.

[9] Rives J, Pire JC, Flament JB, Palot JP, Body C. [Treatment of large eventrations. New therapeutic indications apropos of 322 cases]. *Chirurgie.* 1985;111(3):215-25.

[10] Stoppa RE. The treatment of complicated groin and incisional hernias. *World J Surg.* 1989 Sep-Oct;13(5):545-54.

[11] Read RC. Milestones in the history of hernia surgery: prosthetic repair. *Hernia.* 2004 Feb;8(1):8-14.
[12] LeBlanc KA, Booth WV. Laparoscopic repair of incisional abdominal hernias using expanded polytetrafluoroethylene: preliminary findings. *Surg Laparosc Endosc.* 1993 Feb;3(1):39-41.
[13] Ramirez OM, Ruas E, Dellon AL. "Components separation" method for closure of abdominal-wall defects: an anatomic and clinical study. *Plast Reconstr Surg.* 1990 Sep;86(3):519-26.
[14] Losanoff JE, Basson MD, Laker S, Weiner M, Webber JD, Gruber SA. Subxiphoid incisional hernias after median sternotomy. *Hernia.* 2007 Dec;11(6):473-9.
[15] Dubay DA, Wang X, Kuhn MA, Robson MC, Franz MG. The prevention of incisional hernia formation using a delayed-release polymer of basic fibroblast growth factor. *Ann Surg.* 2004 Jul;240(1):179-86.
[16] Klinge U, Si ZY, Zheng H, Schumpelick V, Bhardwaj RS, Klosterhalfen B. Collagen I/III and matrix metalloproteinases (MMP) 1 and 13 in the fascia of patients with incisional hernias. *J Invest Surg.* 2001 Jan-Feb;14(1):47-54.
[17] Di Vita G, Patti R, D'Agostino P, Caruso G, Arcara M, Buscemi S, et al. Cytokines and growth factors in wound drainage fluid from patients undergoing incisional hernia repair. *Wound Repair Regen.* 2006 May-Jun;14(3):259-64.
[18] Franz MG, Kuhn MA, Nguyen K, Wang X, Ko F, Wright TE, et al. Transforming growth factor beta(2) lowers the incidence of incisional hernias. *J Surg Res.* 2001 May 15;97(2):109-16.
[19] Sahlin S, Ahlberg J, Granstrom L, Ljungstrom KG. Monofilament versus multifilament absorbable sutures for abdominal closure. *Br J Surg.* 1993 Mar;80(3):322-4.
[20] Richards PC, Balch CM, Aldrete JS. Abdominal wound closure. A randomized prospective study of 571 patients comparing continuous vs. interrupted suture techniques. *Ann Surg.* 1983 Feb;197(2):238-43.
[21] Luijendijk RW, Hop WC, van den Tol MP, de Lange DC, Braaksma MM, JN IJ, et al. A comparison of suture repair with mesh repair for incisional hernia. *N Engl J Med.* 2000 Aug 10;343(6):392-8.
[22] Burger JW, Luijendijk RW, Hop WC, Halm JA, Verdaasdonk EG, Jeekel J. Long-term follow-up of a randomized controlled trial of suture versus mesh repair of incisional hernia. *Ann Surg.* 2004 Oct;240(4):578-83; discussion 83-5.

[23] Patton JH, Jr., Berry S, Kralovich KA. Use of human acellular dermal matrix in complex and contaminated abdominal wall reconstructions. *Am J Surg.* 2007 Mar;193(3):360-3; discussion 3.
[24] Hawn MT, Snyder CW, Graham LA, Gray SH, Finan KR, Vick CC. Long-term follow-up of technical outcomes for incisional hernia repair. *J Am Coll Surg.* May;210(5):648-55, 55-7.
[25] Williams RF, Martin DF, Mulrooney MT, Voeller GR. Intraperitoneal modification of the Rives-Stoppa repair for large incisional hernias. *Hernia.* 2008 Apr;12(2):141-5.
[26] Gillion JF, Begin GF, Marecos C, Fourtanier G. Expanded polytetrafluoroethylene patches used in the intraperitoneal or extraperitoneal position for repair of incisional hernias of the anterolateral abdominal wall. *Am J Surg.* 1997 Jul;174(1):16-9.
[27] Franklin ME, Jr., Gonzalez JJ, Jr., Glass JL, Manjarrez A. Laparoscopic ventral and incisional hernia repair: an 11-year experience. *Hernia.* 2004 Feb;8(1):23-7.
[28] Carbajo MA, Martin del Olmo JC, Blanco JI, de la Cuesta C, Toledano M, Martin F, et al. Laparoscopic treatment vs open surgery in the solution of major incisional and abdominal wall hernias with mesh. *Surg Endosc.* 1999 Mar;13(3):250-2.
[29] Misra MC, Bansal VK, Kulkarni MP, Pawar DK. Comparison of laparoscopic and open repair of incisional and primary ventral hernia: results of a prospective randomized study. *Surg Endosc.* 2006 Dec;20(12):1839-45.
[30] Barbaros U, Asoglu O, Seven R, Erbil Y, Dinccag A, Deveci U, et al. The comparison of laparoscopic and open ventral hernia repairs: a prospective randomized study. *Hernia.* 2007 Feb;11(1):51-6.
[31] Pierce RA, Spitler JA, Frisella MM, Matthews BD, Brunt LM. Pooled data analysis of laparoscopic vs. open ventral hernia repair: 14 years of patient data accrual. *Surg Endosc.* 2007 Mar;21(3):378-86.
[32] Cheng H, Rupprecht F, Jackson D, Berg T, Seelig MH. Decision analysis model of incisional hernia after open abdominal surgery. *Hernia.* 2007 Apr;11(2):129-37.
[33] Forbes SS, Eskicioglu C, McLeod RS, Okrainec A. Meta-analysis of randomized controlled trials comparing open and laparoscopic ventral and incisional hernia repair with mesh. *Br J Surg.* 2009 Aug;96(8):851-8.
[34] Rudmik LR, Schieman C, Dixon E, Debru E. Laparoscopic incisional hernia repair: a review of the literature. *Hernia.* 2006 Apr;10(2):110-9.

[35] Goodney PP, Birkmeyer CM, Birkmeyer JD. Short-term outcomes of laparoscopic and open ventral hernia repair: a meta-analysis. *Arch Surg.* 2002 Oct;137(10):1161-5.

[36] Hope WW, Lincourt AE, Newcomb WL, Schmelzer TM, Kercher KW, Heniford BT. Comparing quality-of-life outcomes in symptomatic patients undergoing laparoscopic or open ventral hernia repair. *J Laparoendosc Adv Surg Tech A.* 2008 Aug;18(4):567-71.

[37] Voyles CR, Richardson JD, Bland KI, Tobin GR, Flint LM, Polk HC, Jr. Emergency abdominal wall reconstruction with polypropylene mesh: short-term benefits versus long-term complications. *Ann Surg.* 1981 Aug;194(2):219-23.

[38] Geisler DJ, Reilly JC, Vaughan SG, Glennon EJ, Kondylis PD. Safety and outcome of use of nonabsorbable mesh for repair of fascial defects in the presence of open bowel. *Dis Colon Rectum.* 2003 Aug;46(8):1118-23.

[39] Shah RH, Sharma A, Khullar R, Soni V, Baijal M, Chowbey PK. Laparoscopic repair of incarcerated ventral abdominal wall hernias. *Hernia.* 2008 Oct;12(5):457-63.

[40] Diaz JJ, Jr., Guy J, Berkes MB, Guillamondegui O, Miller RS. Acellular dermal allograft for ventral hernia repair in the compromised surgical field. *Am Surg.* 2006 Dec;72(12):1181-7; discussion 7-8.

[41] Eriksen JR, Gogenur I, Rosenberg J. Choice of mesh for laparoscopic ventral hernia repair. *Hernia.* 2007 Dec;11(6):481-92.

[42] Chelala E, Debardemaeker Y, Elias B, Charara F, Dessily M, Alle JL. Eighty-five redo surgeries after 733 laparoscopic treatments for ventral and incisional hernia: adhesion and recurrence analysis. *Hernia.* Apr;14(2):123-9.

[43] Rauth TP, Poulose BK, Nanney LB, Holzman MD. A comparative analysis of expanded polytetrafluoroethylene and small intestinal submucosa--implications for patch repair in ventral herniorrhaphy. *J Surg Res.* 2007 Nov;143(1):43-9.

[44] Silverman RP, Li EN, Holton LH, 3rd, Sawan KT, Goldberg NH. Ventral hernia repair using allogenic acellular dermal matrix in a swine model. *Hernia.* 2004 Dec;8(4):336-42.

[45] Espinosa-de-los-Monteros A, de la Torre JI, Marrero I, Andrades P, Davis MR, Vasconez LO. Utilization of human cadaveric acellular dermis for abdominal hernia reconstruction. *Ann Plast Surg.* 2007 Mar;58 (3):264-7.

[46] Candage R, Jones K, Luchette FA, Sinacore JM, Vandevender D, Reed RL, 2nd. Use of human acellular dermal matrix for hernia repair: friend or foe? *Surgery.* 2008 Oct;144(4):703-9; discussion 9-11.

[47] Sandor M, Xu H, Connor J, Lombardi J, Harper JR, Silverman RP, et al. Host response to implanted porcine-derived biologic materials in a primate model of abdominal wall repair. *Tissue Eng Part A.* 2008 Dec;14(12):2021-31.

[48] Jarman-Smith ML, Bodamyali T, Stevens C, Howell JA, Horrocks M, Chaudhuri JB. Porcine collagen crosslinking, degradation and its capability for fibroblast adhesion and proliferation. *J Mater Sci Mater Med.* 2004 Aug;15(8):925-32.

[49] Liang HC, Chang Y, Hsu CK, Lee MH, Sung HW. Effects of cross-linking degree of an acellular biological tissue on its tissue regeneration pattern. *Bioaterials.* 2004 Aug;25(17):3541-52.

[50] Rosen MJ. Biologic mesh for abdominal wall reconstruction: a critical appraisal. *Am Surg.* Jan;76(1):1-6.

[51] Breuing K, Butler CE, Ferzoco S, Franz M, Hultman CS, Kilbridge JF, et al. Incisional ventral hernias: review of the literature and recommendations regarding the grading and technique of repair. *Surgery.* Sep;148(3):544-58.

[52] Fabian TC, Croce MA, Pritchard FE, Minard G, Hickerson WL, Howell RL, et al. Planned ventral hernia. Staged management for acute abdominal wall defects. *Ann Surg.* 1994 Jun;219(6):643-50; discussion 51-3.

[53] de Vries Reilingh TS, van Goor H, Rosman C, Bemelmans MH, de Jong D, van Nieuwenhoven EJ, et al. "Components separation technique" for the repair of large abdominal wall hernias. *J Am Coll Surg.* 2003 Jan;196(1):32-7.

[54] Maas SM, van Engeland M, Leeksma NG, Bleichrodt RP. A modification of the "components separation" technique for closure of abdominal wall defects in the presence of an enterostomy. *J Am Coll Surg.* 1999 Jul;189(1):138-40.

[55] Lowe JB, Garza JR, Bowman JL, Rohrich RJ, Strodel WE. Endoscopically assisted "components separation" for closure of abdominal wall defects. *Plast Reconstr Surg.* 2000 Feb;105(2):720-9; quiz 30.

[56] Maas SM, de Vries RS, van Goor H, de Jong D, Bleichrodt RP. Endoscopically assisted "components separation technique" for the repair of complicated ventral hernias. *J Am Coll Surg.* 2002 Mar;194(3):388-90.

[57] Rosen MJ, Williams C, Jin J, McGee MF, Schomisch S, Marks J, et al. Laparoscopic versus open-component separation: a comparative analysis in a porcine model. *Am J Surg.* 2007 Sep;194(3):385-9.

[58] Rosen MJ, Jin J, McGee MF, Williams C, Marks J, Ponsky JL. Laparoscopic component separation in the single-stage treatment of infected abdominal wall prosthetic removal. *Hernia.* 2007 Oct;11(5):435-40.

[59] Ko JH, Wang EC, Salvay DM, Paul BC, Dumanian GA. Abdominal wall reconstruction: lessons learned from 200 "components separation" procedures. *Arch Surg.* 2009 Nov;144(11):1047-55.

[60] Bachman SL, Ramaswamy A, Ramshaw BJ. Early results of midline hernia repair using a minimally invasive component separation technique. *Am Surg.* 2009 Jul;75(7):572-7; discussion 7-8.

[61] Malik K, Bowers SP, Smith CD, Asbun H, Preissler S. A case series of laparoscopic components separation and rectus medialization with laparoscopic ventral hernia repair. *J Laparoendosc Adv Surg Tech A.* 2009 Oct;19(5):607-10.

[62] Witkowski P, Abbonante F, Fedorov I, Sledzinski Z, Pejcic V, Slavin L, et al. Are mesh anchoring sutures necessary in ventral hernioplasty? Multicenter study. *Hernia.* 2007 Dec;11(6):501-8.

[63] Melman L, Jenkins ED, Deeken CR, Brodt MD, Brown SR, Brunt LM, et al. Evaluation of Acute Fixation Strength for Mechanical Tacking Devices and Fibrin Sealant Versus Polypropylene Suture for Laparoscopic Ventral Hernia Repair. *Surg Innov.* Sep 3.

[64] Eriksen JR, Bech JI, Linnemann D, Rosenberg J. Laparoscopic intraperitoneal mesh fixation with fibrin sealant (Tisseel) vs. titanium tacks: a randomised controlled experimental study in pigs. *Hernia.* 2008 Oct;12(5):483-91.

[65] Perrone JM, Soper NJ, Eagon JC, Klingensmith ME, Aft RL, Frisella MM, et al. Perioperative outcomes and complications of laparoscopic ventral hernia repair. *Surgery.* 2005 Oct;138(4):708-15; discussion 15-6.

Chapter 10

Spigelian Hernias

David A. Klima, Igor Belyansky,
Victor B. Tsirline and B. Todd Heniford[*]
Division of Gastrointestinal and Minimally Invasive Surgery,
Department of Surgery, Carolinas Medical Center,
Charlotte, NC, USA

Abstract

A Spigelian hernia is a congenital or acquired defect in the spigelian aponeurosis of anterior abdominal wall. It is present in up to 2% of the population with hernia defects and is most commonly seen in the fourth to seventh decade of life. This aponeurosis is located between the semilunar line (laterally) and the lateral edge of the rectus muscle (medially). This defect is most commonly found in the spigelian belt which is a 6 cm area superior to a line between the anterior superior iliac spines and below the arcuate line. Greater omentum is usually seen incarcerated between the muscles of the lateral abdominal wall and is oftentimes difficult to appreciate on physical exam. These are usually smaller sized defects and thus the

---

[*] Corresponding Author: B. Todd Heniford, MD, Carolinas Laparoscopic and Advanced Surgery Program, Division of GI and Minimally Invasive Surgery, Department of General Surgery, Carolinas Medical Center, 1025 Morehead Medical Plaza, Suite #300, Charlotte, NC 28204, 704-355-3168 (Office), 704-355-5619 (Fax), todd.heniford@carolinashealthcare.org

danger comes when the patient has an incarcerated or strangulated section of small or large bowel. Diagnosis of Spigelian hernias is via Computed Tomography scans, ultrasound or at the time of surgery for a small bowel obstruction or peritonitis. The key to diagnosis is clinical suspicion as well as a thorough history, physical exam and appropriate work-up. Surgical treatment has traditionally been performed through an open approach with a primary closure of the fascia or placement of mesh. More recently, surgeons have demonstrated that both the diagnosis and repair of these hernias can be accomplished laparoscopically with minimal morbidity. Both techniques reportedly have very low recurrence rates and patients with these hernias tend to do well.

Introduction

Spigelian hernias are a rare congenital/acquired abdominal wall defect located in the Spigelian aponeurosis that contains a peritoneal sac, organ or pre-peritoneal fat. Spigelian hernias represent 1-2% of all hernias and can often be overlooked due to its rarity [1]. While few in numbers, with just over one-thousand reported in the literature, it is the most common spontaneous lateral abdominal wall abnormality. Repair of the defect can be performed from both an open as well as laparoscopic approach depending on the surgeon's familiarity and expertise. The importance in the understanding and early diagnosis of this condition lies with its high incarceration rate estimated at 17-40% [1-3].

The history of the Spigelian hernia began in the 1600's and our knowledge has continued to evolve into the early 21st century. The Belgian anatomist Adriaan van der Spieghel was the first to describe the semilunar line in 1645 [4-6]. It was not until almost 100 years later that Henri Francois Le Dran described a "rupture" along this line in 1742 [1, 4, 6]. Josef Klinkosch was the first to use the term "Spigelian hernia" and describe the hernia as a defect along the semilunar line [7, 8]. Interestingly, the first case reported in the literature was in a child in 1935 by Scopinaro, but since that time greater than 90% of cases reported have been in adults [9]. Most commonly the patients present in their sixth decade of life. While some individual studies state an increased etiology on the left side or in females [9], there seems to be no predominant side or gender and approximately 3% of them present bilaterally [2].

Anatomy

The Spigelian aponeurosis is the aponeurotic band of the transversus abdominus muscle that is bordered laterally by the semilunar line and medially by the lateral edge of the rectus muscle [1, 4-6]. The semilunar lines occur bilaterally and represent the transition of the transversus abdominus from muscle to aponeurosis. These lines course from the costochondral junction of the inferior edge of the ninth rib down to the pubic spine inferiorly. Above the arcuate line, also known as the line of Douglas or semicircular line, the internal oblique aponeurosis splits around the rectus muscle, joining the Spigelian aponeurosis posteriorly to form the posterior rectus sheath and the external oblique aponeurosis anteriorly to form the anterior rectus sheath. Below the arcuate line, the posterior structures merge anteriorly leaving only the peritoneum posterior to the rectus muscle (Figure 1).

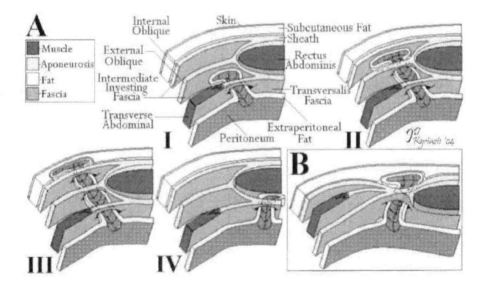

Figure 1. A three dimensional schematic representation of the types of Spigelian hernias. Spigelian hernia is shown at two different levels: A. Above the arcuate line and B. Below the arcuate line. For hernias above the arcuate line, there are four types: I. Through the transversalis fascia, but posterior to the internal oblique; II. Through the tranversalis fascia and internal oblique, but deep to the external oblique; III. Through all three fascial layers. IV. Penetrating the posterior rectus sheath. (Printed with permission from J. David Richardson, Editor-in-Chief of The American Surgeon; Skandalakis, et al, 2006).

The Spigelian hernia belt is the area where a majority of hernias occur [1, 4, 6]. This area is an approximately 6 cm band that traverses the Spigelian fascia from the umbilicus to the anterior superior iliac spines (ASIS). In the middle of this region lies the arcuate line where the fibers split from a single unified layer inferiorly into the anterior and posterior layers superiorly. At this junction is where the lateral abdominal wall is at its weakest. The five different types of Spigelian hernias demonstrated in Figure 1 are dependant on their anatomical location along the abdomen and fascial layers through which they penetrate. Oftentimes the overlying external oblique and fascia remain intact after herniation, leading to compression of the contents within the hernia sac. Only 2 - 18% of patients have a subcutaneously located hernia sac, making the ability to define the mass and palpate a defect much more difficult [1-3].

Etiology

The etiology is oftentimes debated and over the years multiple theories have accumulated. The earliest theory was that by Sir Ashley Cooper [4, 10, 11]. He suggested the "vascular theory," which stated that these hernias prolapse through small defects in the fascia secondary to perforating vessels. Similarly, Thevenot and Gabourd suggested that the defect was formed by the perforation of the inferior epigastric artery through the transversalis fascia [12]. Read and others subsequently challenged this theory with the observation that vessels were rarely seen passing through the defect and that Spigelian hernias are seen at multiple sites along the spigelian aponeurosis [13, 14].

A second, more accepted theory is the musculoaponeurotic defect theory. Zimmerman and River both noted that the transversus abdominal aponeurosis frequently contained defects [4, 15]. It was hypothesized that these defects give way to small pieces of preperitoneal fat and omentum, which leads to a progressive enlargement of the defect with a lead point for subsequent herniation. Co-morbidities such as morbid obesity, connective tissue disorders, aging and chronic obstructive pulmonary disease (COPD) have been demonstrated to be predisposing factors for abdominal wall defects and may contribute to this theory. Mersheimer felt that the most important factor is that the angle of the aponeurotic fibers of the transverse abdominis and internal oblique form a gridiron superiorly, leading to a stonger abdominal wall [16]. Inferiorly, below the umbilicus, the fibers run parallel, making this area much weaker and more prone to herniation

[16]. Another predisposing factor is previous abdominal surgery. Incisional hernias occur at a rate of 3-20% after laparotomy depending on a variety of factors including obesity, wound infection and location [3, 17, 18].

Spigelian hernias in the pediatric age group have often been considered congenital. This thought has been challenged in pediatric patients presenting at an older age as well as the large proportion of patients that present as adults (>95%) [4]. A definition of congenital anomaly includes those changes that are present at birth. White reported that nine of the 30 reported pediatric cases were noted from birth and felt to be congenital in nature [19]. He noted an inherent failure of fusion where the semilunar line and semicircular line of Douglas crossed with a well defined rim of defect [19]. Interestingly, the embryogenesis of the abdomen is different above the umbilicus as compared to that below the umbilicus [4]. In the supraumbilical area, the intercostal and abdominal muscles form from the merging of the thoracic somites with the somatopleura. Below the umbilicus, the mesenchyme comes from many sources including the umbilical ring and the caudal eminence [4]. This provides a closure of the inferior abdominal wall prior to the migration of the myotome, thus giving us the arcuate line with complete mesodermal fusion by the 12th week. Interestingly, 19% of pediatric cases have ipsilateral undescended testes and up to 35% of patients have other congenital anomalies [20]. The association between abdominal wall defects and cryptorchidism is often attributed to a lack of abdominal pressure in the abdomen resulting in undescended testes [21].

Overall, our impression is that a combined theory offers the most likely explanation. Early presentations such as those present at birth are congenital in origin by definition. While the vascular theory is less likely, small perforations in the transverse abdominus aponeurosis may occasionally be the source. Many people may have certain genetic predispositions to herniation including a congenital defect or weakening of the abdominal wall. These factors combined with trauma, obesity, or multiple pregnancies that distort the abdominal musculature may lead to further weakening of the abdominal wall, predisposing people for herniation.

Presentation

The presentation of these patients can be varied and oftentimes difficult to discern. The most common presenting symptoms are a palpable mass, vague abdominal pain or a combination of both. Other presentations include obstruction, peritonitis and up to 3% of patients can be entirely asymptomatic. Physical exam can be unreliable since as few as 31% of patients have a palpable abdominal mass on physical exam which leads to the logical conclusion that these hernias are likely underreported [2]. In the largest series of Spigelian hernia repairs to date, palpable mass was the most common presentation, but Larson reported that only 64% of patients had a definable abnormality on physical examination [2]. This leaves 36% of patients without the appropriate diagnosis based on physical exam alone. In the study by Artioukh, only 53% of the repairs had a suspected Spigelian hernia pre-operatively [3] consistent with earlier reports [14]. One differentiating feature of these hernias is the worsening of pain upon standing due to the stretching of the abdominal wall, which oftentimes resolves upon lying down. Many times these hernias are mistaken pre-operatively for an inguinal hernia when found very low, colon mass, appendiceal mass or even diverticulitis [22-27]. This can lead to difficulty in preoperative decision making, but the more recent use of laparoscopy as well as technologic advances can supplement the physical exam and help avoid the large midline incision associated with an exploratory laparotomy.

The importance of early diagnosis of Spigelian hernias lies in the high incarceration rate, ranging from 17-24%. This is most likely secondary to the small defect size as well as the sharp fascial edges [2, 3, 13]. Average defect size is 0.5-2.0 cm in diameter, although some have been described as large as 10 cm [28, 29]. Literature reports include multiple organs of incarceration including the stomach, small bowel, omentum, cecum, sigmoid, bladder, Meckel's diverticulum, gallbladder, testicle and appendix [5, 30-34]. Patients have even presented with appendicitis secondary to incarceration [33, 35].

Diagnosis

Due to the difficulty in diagnosing Spigelian hernias with history and physical exam, imaging has become an important part of the pre-operative work-up. Ultrasound has shown itself to be a useful screening tool when the diagnosis is questionable. Sonographic evaluation of the Spigelian belt may be the best technique, using lateral sweeps starting at the lateral edge of the rectus. Accuracy when utilizing ultrasound has been demonstrated to be as high as 79% [5, 36]. The ultrasonographic signs for making the diagnosis of Spigelian hernia are: 1) interruption of the deepest layer of peritoneum and preperitoneal fat in transverse scans, 2) demonstration of a hernial orifice in the spigelian aponeurosis, 3) intramurally located sac, and 4) sac contents in the form of intestine or omentum [1]. Ultrasound is aided by the well-defined aponeurosis present at the orifice which allows for differentiation between the bowel wall and defect. Torzilli suggested that modern ultrasound not only allows for an accurate diagnosis of a Spigelian hernia, but demonstrates changes in the abdominal wall and hernia sac with inspiration and standing [37]. This gives the surgeon an interactive approach to diagnosis at a reasonable cost and the opportunity to intervene and avoid an emergent operation via reduction of the hernia [38]. But, of course, this depends on the quality of the ultrasound and its reading, which can be variable when technicians and physicians do not have great experience looking at the abdominal wall.

Computed Tomography (CT) scans have become increasingly more popular over the last 20 years and have helped establish the diagnosis pre-operatively in a majority of patients. While it does not give one the flexibility of positional changes and interactive reduction, CT does have multiple advantages over sonography. First, it can correctly diagnose a hernia defect in patients in whom a Spigelian hernia was not expected or in patients without a palpable mass of undetermined etiology on physical exam (Figure 2) [39]. Secondly, the organ of incarceration can easily be determined as can the exact location of the hernia sac [40]. If the hernia sac contains only fat, a lipoma of the abdominal wall should be entertained in the differential. Thirdly, any signs of bowel necrosis or obstruction can be diagnosed so appropriate resuscitation and nasogastric decompression can take place prior to surgery. Larson's experience in 76 patients used CT scans in only 25% of patients [2]. Thirteen of the 19 scans obtained were positive for Spigelian hernia rendering a sensitivity of only 68%. Shenouda and others have demonstrated the effectiveness of utilizing CT in 3 cases where the diagnosis was questionable [41]. Each scan demonstrated the abdominal wall defect clearly as well as the hernia contents [30]. Lastly, CT allows for other intra-abdominal pathology to be investigated and ruled out pre-operatively [23, 28, 30, 31].

Roentgenography is also a consideration in establishing the correct diagnosis. A palpable mass should be present since a plain film or contrast study will not delineate the borders of the hernia. If a colonic incarceration is expected, barium enema may be useful. For small bowel incarceration, patients may have an x-ray consistent with small bowel obstruction with multiple air-fluid levels and dilated small bowel loops. Small bowel follow-through can help delineate the location along the small intestine, but once again, confirms only the obstruction and not the hernia itself.

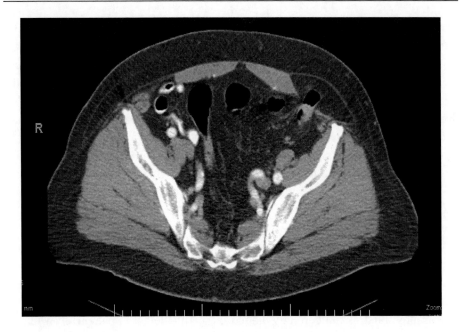

Figure 2. Computed Tomography scan demonstrating a left sided Spigelian hernia.

In patients without an incarceration or a palpable mass, roentgenography has a minimal role. Some have suggested that herniography can be used for inguinal, femoral and obturator hernias, which may have a similar presentation. For those patients in whom the surgeon has a high suspicion of Spigelian hernia, due to the sensitivity and specificity of other diagnostic tests, herniography has limited use [42].

Mills and Selinkoff suggest that anyone with well localized pain in the appropriate location should undergo surgical exploration [8]. Artioukh used this technique on nine patients and confirmed Spigelian hernia in seven, with one inguinal hernia and one without any demonstratable abnormality [3, 8]. Now, with the emergence of minimally invasive procedures, many times these are found on diagnostic laparoscopy and repaired at the same setting.

In summary, the diagnosis of Spigelian hernia can often be difficult to ascertain on physical exam alone. This can be due to the small defect, obese population, low clinical suspicion and compression by the intact external oblique. X-rays and herniography have little use in these patients. Ultrasound can be used when the examiner has significant experience with this tool and can provide interactive confirmation of the hernia. CT is very effective at delineating the defect size, location as well as concomitant obstruction and should be utilized in those patients in whom a diagnosis is unknown, which can be common. It is important to keep in mind that none of these diagnostic tests are 100% sensitive, and that many times, the diagnosis is not confirmed until the time of surgery.

Surgical Repair

Treatment for a newly diagnosed Spigelian hernia is surgery, especially given their tendency to incarcerate. Repair can be performed either by the traditional open approach or via a laparoscopic technique. Open repair has most commonly been accomplished with a transverse incision and primary repair [1, 2, 5, 42-45], although most hernias are now repaired with mesh. The hernia is most commonly encountered when incising the anterior rectus sheath and/or the external oblique aponeurosis. The hernia is then reduced and the posterior fascia is then closed with suture as is the external oblique aponeurosis. A synthetic mesh underlay or onlay can be accomplished either before or after closure of the muscle and fascia. If the bowel is strangulated, carrying the fascial incision medially to release the hernia contents may help facilitate reduction. If bowel is compromised, small bowel resection and reanastamosis can be performed through the same defect. It is important to note, that some Spigelian hernias can present posterior to the rectus muscle, thus a more medial dissection to expose this area of the posterior rectus sheath may be warranted [1]. This approach can be compromised when the pre-operative diagnosis is unclear, so at times a midline laparotomy will have been or may need to be performed [46]. The advantages to this approach are that the surgeon can explore the peritoneum for any evidence of other defects and make sure any incarcerated bowel is viable.

There are reports describing that mesh may not be as strongly indicated in the repair of these defects as most others in the abdominal wall. Hsieh et. al. reported their data on open Spigelian hernia repairs using mesh in four and no mesh in seven patients [46]. There were no recurrences in either group after an average follow-up of at least 6 years. All three of Larson's recurrences were in the group without mesh, but only five of the 76 patients received mesh at the initial operation [2]. Sanchez-Montes described a new open technique using a preshaped polypropylene umbrella-type plug [47]. This mesh was sutured to the adjacent tissues and the external oblique was closed over the plug. They reported no recurrences at a minimum of 1 year of follow-up. Mouton described his experience with 35 open Spigelian hernia repairs. In 14 cases, a pre-peritoneal nonresorbable mesh was placed electively when the fascial tissues were considered of "weak quality." There were three radiological recurrences, all within the group without mesh. We are currently aware of only 12 reported recurrences in the literature and none of them have occurred after the placement of mesh [2, 45]. This recurrence data, however, may be underreported due to the lack of long-term follow-up.

The first reported case of laparoscopic ventral hernia repair was performed by LeBlanc in 1991 [48]. Shortly thereafter, the first laparoscopic Spigelian hernia repair was performed by Carter only a year later [49]. Since that time, multiple small case reports have been published looking at the effectiveness and difficulty of this repair. Moreno-Egea et al reported the only randomized prospective trial looking at laparoscopic versus open repair of Spigelian hernias [50]. No significant differences in recurrence between the two groups after an average 3.5 year follow-up were noted. Significant differences in hospital length of stay (5 days versus 1 day) and morbidities led to their conclusion that laparoscopic repair with mesh was superior to open repair. One of the major limitations of this study though was that the laparoscopic approach was not standardized. Mesh was placed in the intra-abdominal position in three patients, while the other eight received a total extraperitoneal repair (TEP). Three case series have looked at laparoscopic repair with good success. Mittal performed six intraperitoneal repairs, two transabdominal pre-peritoneal repairs (TAPP) and two TEP's [13]. They reported no recurrences or mesh infections with a mean follow-up of greater than 3 years. Similarly, Palanivelu and colleagues repaired eight Spigelian hernias with suture repair of the defect and intraperitoneal placement of mesh [51]. Once again, there were no post-operative complications or recurrences. Finally, Patle et al and Saber et al each performed laparoscopic repair in six consecutive patients (total of 12) without recurrence or complication [52, 53].

For the surgeon skilled in laparoscopy, the TAPP and intraperitoneal approach gives one the ability to survey the entire abdomen when the diagnosis is uncertain and clearly define the aponeurotic defect. After identification of the hernia, two or three additional ports are placed in the abdomen and the hernia is reduced. In the intraperitoneal approach, an ePTFE or composite mesh with an anti-adhesive barrier is placed in the abdomen at this time using the scroll technique previously described [54]. The mesh is then unfurled and sutured to the abdominal wall with a suture passer; tacks are next added to fill in the gaps between sutures to prevent internal herniation between sutures. Additional, intermittent sutures are added as needed. Usually we look for at least 4 cm of overlap [54], but there are no scientific studies that factually back these numbers up. In the TAPP approach, after reduction of the hernia, the peritoneum is incised and peeled away from the abdominal wall [13]. This allows for placement of the mesh in the preperitoneal space and thus a non-coated or unprotected mesh is applicable. The mesh is is sutured and tacked in position, and the peritoneum is reapproximated to the abdominal wall using clips or tacks.

The TEP approach ideally never breaks through the peritoneum. After entering into the pre-peritoneal space, a balloon is inserted and inflated to expand this potential space [13]. The steps mentioned above for TAPP are repeated for the placement of the mesh. The main advantage to TEP is that there is no entry into the abdominal cavity and no need for peritoneal closure after mesh placement. One of the disadvantages of this technique, however, is the inability to explore the abdomen and address other intra-abdominal pathology if indicated.

Overall, numerous studies have demonstrated the benefits of laparoscopy in ventral hernia repairs. The major advantage is a decreased risk of infection. A recent meta-analysis by Forbes looking at laparoscopic versus open ventral hernia repairs demonstrated there were no differences in recurrence, but the patients undergoing laparoscopic repair had a shorter length of stay and fewer wound infections [55]. Other advantages demonstrated in similar studies include a shorter recovery time and improved postoperative cosmesis [56, 57]. In the study by Moreno-Agea, patients went home almost 4 days earlier with the laparoscopic repair [50]. Whether performed open or laparoscopically, operative treatment of Spigelian hernias most often result in a quality repair with minimal morbidity. Therefore, patient preference and surgeon expertise may weigh heavily on the choice of individual repair.

Special Considerations

Low-lying Spigelian hernias are a special type of hernia that present with signs and symptoms that can easily be confused with inguinal hernias. Physical exam may reveal pain and a palpable mass in the anterior abdominal wall with varying symptoms depending on the content of the hernia sac which most commonly contains preperitoneal fat [1, 58]. The incidence of low-lying Spigelian hernias may be underestimated due to the similar presentation and decreased awareness. Pre-operative diagnosis can once again be defined by ultrasound or CT scan, but most patients with inguinal hernias do not usually receive further pre-operative work-up or diagnostic imaging. Klimopoulos was able to appropriately diagnose a Spigelian hernia on physical exam alone in 15 of 26 patients, but duplication of these results have not been confirmed [58]. Repair for the low Spigelian hernia has been described with and without mesh [58]. Once again, if the diagnosis is not confirmed pre-operatively, laparoscopic exploration and repair is similar to that for an inguinal hernia with the preperitoneal placement of mesh either via TAPP or TEP.

Conclusion

Spigelian hernias are a rare, but important form of hernia secondary to its variable presentation, difficult diagnosis and high incidence of incarceration on presentation. The etiology of these hernias is multifactorial and most likely has a congenital weakening that predisposes one to herniation after increased abdominal pressure (obesity), poor respiratory status (COPD), surgery or multiple pregnancies altering the contour and fascia of the abdominal wall. Physical exam can be unreliable and often needs supplementation via diagnostic imaging. Ultrasound in patients with a definable bulge on their anterior abdominal wall allows for an interactive diagnosis with fair results. Computed Tomography can allow one to define the defect location and hernia contents, but small defects may not be detected if hernia contents have been reduced. Surgical repair is the treatment of choice in these patients. Open primary repair has certainly been reported, but use of mesh has given promising results with no reported mesh infection or recurrences. Laparoscopy allows the advantage of looking throughout the abdomen for other suspected pathology in a patient with an undefined etiology. Repair is usually very successful regardless of approach. Because of this, the surgeon's familiarity and patient's preference usually dictate the best approach.

References

[1] Spangen, L., Spigelian hernia. *World J Surg*, 1989. 13(5): p. 573-80.
[2] Larson, D.W. and D.R. Farley, Spigelian hernias: repair and outcome for 81 patients. *World J Surg*, 2002. 26(10): p. 1277-81.
[3] Artioukh, D.Y. and S.J. Walker, Spigelian herniae: presentation, diagnosis and treatment. *J R Coll Surg Edinb*, 1996. 41(4): p. 241-3.

[4] Skandalakis, P.N., et al., Spigelian hernia: surgical anatomy, embryology, and technique of repair. *Am Surg*, 2006. 72(1): p. 42-8.
[5] Spangen, L., Spigelian hernia. *Surg Clin North Am*, 1984. 64(2): p. 351-66.
[6] Singer, J.A. and A.R. Mansberger, Jr., Spigelian hernia. *Arch Surg*, 1973. 107(4): p. 515-7.
[7] Amendolara, M., Videolaparoscopic treatment of Spigelian hernias. *Surg Laparosc Endosc*, 1998. 8(2): p. 136-9.
[8] Mills, J.L. and P.M. Selinkoff, Spigelian hernia: uncommon or unrecognized? *South Med J*, 1985. 78(4): p. 411-3.
[9] de la Hermosa, A.R., Prats, I.A., Liendo, P.M., Noboa, F.N., Calero, A.M., Spigelian hernia. *Personal experience and review of the literature. Revista Espanola de Enfermedades Digestivas*, 2010. 102: p. 583-586.
[10] Robinson, H.B., Hernia through the semilunar line. *Br J Surg*, 1914. 2: p. 2.
[11] Cooper, A., ed. *The Anatomy and Surgical Treatment of Inguinal and Congenital Hernia*. 1804, Langman, Hurst, Rees and Orme. London.
[12] Thevenot, T. and T. Gabourd, Les hernies spontanees du repli semi-lunaire de Spiegel. *Rev Chir Paris*, 1907. 35: p. 18.
[13] Mittal, T., et al., Diagnosis and management of Spigelian hernia: A review of literature and our experience. *J Minim Access Surg*, 2008. 4(4): p. 95-98.
[14] Read, R.C., Observations on the etiology of spigelian hernia. *Ann Surg*, 1960. 152: p. 1004-9.
[15] River, L.P., Spigelian Hernia: Spontaneous Lateral Ventral Hernia through the Semilunar Line. *Ann Surg*, 1942. 116(3): p. 405-11.
[16] Leis, H.P., Jr., W.L. Mersheimer, and J.M. Winfield, Spontaneous lateral ventral hernia; spigelian or semilunar hernia. *Surgery*, 1958. 43(2): p. 328-33.
[17] Mudge, M. and L.E. Hughes, Incisional hernia: a 10 year prospective study of incidence and attitudes. *Br J Surg*, 1985. 72(1): p. 70-1.
[18] Carlson, M.A., K.A. Ludwig, and R.E. Condon, Ventral hernia and other complications of 1,000 midline incisions. *South Med J*, 1995. 88(4): p. 450-3.
[19] White, J.J., Concomitant Spigelian and inguinal hernias in a neonate. *J Pediatr Surg*, 2002. 37(4): p. 659-60.
[20] Al-Salem, A.H., Congenital spigelian hernia and cryptorchidism: cause or coincidence? *Pediatr Surg Int*, 2000. 16(5-6): p. 433-6.

[21] Levy, G., et al., Pre-operative sonographic diagnosis of incarcerated neonatal Spigelian hernia containing the testis. *Pediatr Radiol*, 2003. 33(6): p. 407-9.
[22] Christianakis, E., et al., Low Spigelian hernia in a 6-year-old boy presenting as an incarcerated inguinal hernia: a case report. *J Med Case Reports*, 2009. 3: p. 34.
[23] Miller, R., O. Lifschitz, and E. Mavor, Incarcerated Spigelian hernia mimicking obstructing colon carcinoma. *Hernia*, 2008. 12(1): p. 87-9.
[24] Losanoff, J.E. and M.D. Basson, Giant Spigelian hernias. *Hernia*, 2007. 11(4): p. 381-2; author reply 383.
[25] Sharma, H., L. Rich, and M.D. Kelly, Spigelian hernia presenting as an appendicular mass. *South Med J*, 2007. 100(10): p. 1037-8.
[26] Delis, N., et al., Incarcerated spigelian hernia mimicking diverticulitis: detection by multidetector computed tomography. *Int J Colorectal Dis*, 2006. 21(8): p. 851-3.
[27] Rogers, F.B. and P.C. Camp, A strangulated Spigelian hernia mimicking diverticulitis. *Hernia*, 2001. 5(1): p. 51-2.
[28] Ribeiro, E.A., R.J. Cruz, Jr., and S.M. Moreira, Intestinal obstruction induced by a giant incarcerated Spigelian hernia: case report and review of the literature. *Sao Paulo Med J*, 2005. 123(3): p. 148-50.
[29] Topal, E., et al., Giant spigelian hernia due to abdominal wall injury: a case report. *Hernia*, 2007. 11(1): p. 67-9.
[30] Gough, V.M. and M. Vella, Timely computed tomography scan diagnoses spigelian hernia: a case study. *Ann R Coll Surg Engl*, 2009. 91(8): p. W9-10.
[31] Habib, E. and A. Elhadad, Spigelian hernia long considered as diverticulitis: CT scan diagnosis and laparoscopic treatment. Computed tomography. *Surg Endosc*, 2003. 17(1): p. 159.
[32] Dixon, E. and J.A. Heine, Incarcerated Meckel's diverticulum in a Spigelian hernia. *Am J Surg*, 2000. 180(2): p. 126.
[33] Lin, P.H., et al., Right lower quadrant abdominal pain due to appendicitis and an incarcerated spigelian hernia. *Am Surg*, 2000. 66(8): p. 725-7.
[34] Jain, K.M., et al., Spigelian hernia. *Am Surg*, 1977. 43(9): p. 596-600.
[35] Carr, J.A. and R. Karmy-Jones, Spigelian hernia with Crohn's appendicitis. *Surg Laparosc Endosc*, 1998. 8(5): p. 398-9.
[36] Nelson, R.L., et al., Ultrasonography of the abdominal wall in the diagnosis of spigelian hernia. *Am Surg*, 1980. 46(7): p. 373-6.

[37] Torzilli, G., et al., The usefulness of ultrasonography in the diagnosis of the Spigelian hernia. *Int Surg,* 1995. 80(3): p. 280-2.
[38] Torzilli, G., et al., Ultrasound-guided reduction of an incarcerated Spigelian hernia. *Ultrasound Med Biol,* 2001. 27(8): p. 1133-5.
[39] Vas, W., K.T. Nguyen, and W.P. Cockshott, Computed tomography diagnosis of Spigelian hernia. Case report. *Diagn Imaging,* 1980. 49(6): p. 326-9.
[40] Balthazar, E.J., B.R. Subramanyam, and A. Megibow, Spigelian hernia: CT and ultrasonography diagnosis. *Gastrointest Radiol,* 1984. 9(1): p. 81-4.
[41] Shenouda, N.F., B.B. Hyams, and M.B. Rosenbloom, Evaluation of Spigelian hernia by CT. *J Comput Assist Tomogr,* 1990. 14(5): p. 777-8.
[42] Gullmo, A., Herniography. *World J Surg,* 1989. 13(5): p. 560-8.
[43] Houlihan, T.J., A review of Spigelian hernias. *Am J Surg,* 1976. 131(6): p. 734-5.
[44] Holder, L.E. and H.J. Schneider, Spigelian hernias: anatomy and roentgenographic manifestations. *Radiology,* 1974. 112(2): p. 309-13.
[45] Mouton, W.G., et al., Preperitoneal mesh repair in Spigelian hernia. *Int Surg,* 2006. 91(5): p. 262-4.
[46] Hsieh, H.F., et al., Spiegelian hernia: mesh or not? *Rev Esp Enferm Dig,* 2007. 99(9): p. 502-4.
[47] Sanchez-Montes, I. and M. Deysine, Spigelian hernias: a new repair technique using preshaped polypropylene umbrella plugs. *Arch Surg,* 1998. 133(6): p. 670-2.
[48] LeBlanc, K., Laparoscopic treatment of ventral hernia. *Surg Endosc,* 2001. 15(10): p. 1242; author reply 1243.
[49] Carter, J.E. and C. Mizes, Laparoscopic diagnosis and repair of spigelian hernia: report of a case and technique. *Am J Obstet Gynecol,* 1992. 167(1): p. 77-8.
[50] Moreno-Egea, A., et al., Open vs laparoscopic repair of spigelian hernia: a prospective randomized trial. *Arch Surg,* 2002. 137(11): p. 1266-8.
[51] Palanivelu, C., et al., Laparoscopic transabdominal preperitoneal repair of spigelian hernia. *JSLS,* 2006. 10(2): p. 193-8.
[52] Saber, A.A., et al., Laparoscopic spigelian hernia repair: the scroll technique. *Am Surg,* 2008. 74(2): p. 108-12.
[53] Patle, N.M., et al., Laparoscopic repair of spigelian hernia: our experience. *J Laparoendosc Adv Surg Tech A,* 2010. 20(2): p. 129-33.

[54] Heniford, B.T., et al., Laparoscopic repair of ventral hernias: nine years' experience with 850 consecutive hernias. *Ann Surg*, 2003. 238(3): p. 391-9; discussion 399-400.
[55] Forbes, S.S., et al., Meta-analysis of randomized controlled trials comparing open and laparoscopic ventral and incisional hernia repair with mesh. *Br J Surg*, 2009. 96(8): p. 851-8.
[56] Misiakos, E.P., et al., Laparoscopic ventral hernia repair: pros and cons compared with open hernia repair. *JSLS*, 2008. 12(2): p. 117-25.
[57] Bedi, A.P., et al., Laparoscopic incisional and ventral hernia repair. *J Minim Access Surg*, 2007. 3(3): p. 83-90.
[58] Klimopoulos, S., et al., Low spigelian hernias: experience of 26 consecutive cases in 24 patients. *Eur J Surg*, 2001. 167(8): p. 631-3.

Index

2

20th century, 143
21st century, 192

A

abdominal wall, viii, xi, xii, 32, 33, 34, 35, 36, 38, 39, 40, 41, 42, 51, 58, 59, 63, 64, 69, 70, 71, 77, 79, 125, 126, 127, 133, 135, 136, 139, 140, 141, 142, 146, 148, 152, 153, 156, 157, 161, 162, 163, 164, 165, 167, 173, 174, 175, 176, 178, 179, 180, 183, 186, 187, 락188, 189, 191, 192, 194, 195, 196, 197, 199, 200, 201, 202, 204
access, 27, 29, 109, 122, 126, 146, 180
acid, 93, 98, 101, 103, 108, 109, 173
adductor, 62
adenocarcinoma, 49
adhesion, 39, 61, 119, 168, 172, 173, 174, 187, 188
adhesions, xii, 39, 41, 42, 43, 52, 76, 118, 120, 124, 140, 152, 154, 174
adjustment, ix, 82, 84, 90, 91
adulthood, 9
adults, xi, 4, 5, 12, 36, 92, 109, 123, 139, 141, 142, 143, 147, 156, 160, 192, 195
advancement, 177
advancements, x, 100, 163, 184
adverse effects, 40, 152
aesthetic, 38
age, ix, xi, 2, 3, 6, 26, 33, 61, 62, 63, 69, 82, 83, 84, 85, 86, 89, 90, 91, 92, 96, 104, 127, 128, 139, 140, 154, 162, 195
airways, 93
alveolar macrophage, 98
anastomosis, 48, 59
anatomy, 37, 165, 203, 205
anchoring, 105, 189
anemia, 75
angiogenesis, 166
antibiotic, 40, 51, 126, 128, 144, 157
antigenicity, 174
anus, 32, 36, 79
aplasia, 83
aponeurosis, xii, 4, 5, 8, 20, 58, 61, 64, 70, 164, 176, 177, 191, 192, 193, 194, 195, 197, 199
appendicitis, 131, 132, 196, 204
arrhythmia, 130, 132
artery, 65, 66, 68, 130, 131, 132, 194

ascites, xi, 59, 63, 139, 141, 144, 148, 159
aspiration, 75, 97, 98
assessment, 20, 35, 77, 95, 109, 146, 171
asthma, 93, 98, 141
asymptomatic, viii, x, 31, 34, 38, 46, 63, 65, 71, 77, 78, 99, 106, 127, 147, 196
atelectasis, 73
atrophy, 11, 24
attachment, 92
audit, 49
authorities, 4, 6
aversion, 91, 92
avoidance, 10, 115
awareness, 73, 201

B

back pain, 142
bacteria, 151
bacterial infection, 136
barium, 197
barium enema, 197
barriers, 162, 163
base, xii, 8, 12, 13, 29, 97, 106, 161
benefits, 12, 43, 144, 145, 149, 170, 187, 201
benign, x, 99
bias, ix, 82, 84, 91
bioavailability, 41
biocompatibility, 174
biomaterials, 43, 44
biopolymers, 174
birth weight, 83, 85, 89
births, 77
bleeding, viii, 32, 75, 171
blood, xi, 38, 126, 128, 133, 134, 135, 137, 149, 176
blood flow, 137
blood supply, 38, 176
blood transfusion, xi, 126, 137
blood transfusions, xi, 126, 137
BMI, 102, 128, 130, 132, 134, 136, 178

body composition, 93
body mass index, xi, 126, 128, 143
bone, 20, 165
bowel, viii, ix, xi, xii, 32, 33, 34, 35, 36, 37, 38, 40, 41, 42, 44, 45, 50, 52, 53, 57, 59, 62, 65, 66, 67, 68, 69, 70, 71, 72, 73, 75, 78, 113, 126, 130, 132, 133, 135, 139, 142, 147, 152, 154, 155, 162, 163, 167, 172, 178, 187, 192, 196, 197, 199
bowel obstruction, viii, ix, xii, xiii, 32, 41, 57, 65, 66, 140, 142, 154, 192, 197
bowel perforation, xi, 126, 132, 133
bowel sounds, 73
brain, 71
breathing, 92, 165, 173
bronchoconstriction, 93, 98
burn, 75, 104
Butcher, 48

C

cadaver, 102
calcium, 103
cancer, 32, 44, 141
capillary, 126, 136, 174
carcinogenesis, 173
carcinoma, 204
cardiac surgery, 137
cardiomyopathy, 146
cardiovascular disease, 141
case study, 204
catheter, 60, 119, 120, 127, 152
cauterization, 118
cecum, 67, 196
cesarean section, 76, 79
challenges, 41, 145, 171, 172
chemical, 175
chemotherapy, 44
Chicago, 4, 84, 128
childhood, vii, 1, 2, 4, 25, 112, 122

Index

children, vii, xi, 1, 2, 3, 4, 5, 6, 7, 8, 9, 10, 11, 12, 13, 14, 15, 16, 17, 19, 20, 21, 24, 25, 26, 27, 28, 29, 58, 84, 89, 93, 94, 95, 96, 97, 98, 112, 115, 118, 121, 122, 123, 124, 139, 140, 142, 147, 155
cholecystectomy, 160
chromosome, 72, 103
chronic illness, 97
chronic obstructive pulmonary disease, xi, 126, 139, 194
cirrhosis, xi, 63, 139, 141, 144, 159
City, 16
clarity, 169
classification, 95, 130, 132
cleavage, 6
clinical assessment, 35
clinical diagnosis, 34
clinical examination, 69, 128
clinical trials, 109
closure, vii, xi, xiii, 1, 8, 9, 11, 13, 14, 17, 25, 28, 39, 60, 61, 74, 83, 92, 105, 110, 112, 115, 116, 117, 119, 121, 123, 124, 127, 130, 131, 133, 135, 136, 137, 140, 144, 145, 149, 150, 151, 153, 155, 158, 162, 163, 167, 170, 171, 175, 176, 179, 181, 185, 188, 192, 195, 199, 201
clothing, 41
CNS, 59
CO2, 152
colic, 65, 66, 67
colitis, 47, 103
collagen, 55, 102, 126, 147, 165, 166, 173, 174, 188
collateral, 149
colon, xi, 34, 44, 52, 61, 64, 66, 67, 68, 72, 75, 79, 131, 139, 142, 196, 204
colonoscopy, 142
color, iv, 7, 128
colostomy, 32, 33, 36, 37, 46, 47, 48, 49, 50, 53, 55, 127
common presenting symptoms, 195
common symptoms, x, 100
community, 109

comparative analysis, 187, 189
compartment syndrome, 127
complexity, 70
compliance, 173
complications, vii, xi, xii, 2, 10, 11, 12, 23, 24, 33, 35, 39, 40, 43, 45, 46, 47, 48, 49, 50, 61, 85, 92, 100, 103, 105, 106, 110, 112, 121, 125, 128, 140, 142, 144, 146, 148, 152, 154, 160, 169, 171, 174, 175, 177, 179, 184, 187, 189, 200, 203
composition, 93
compression, 65, 73, 78, 194, 198
computed tomography, 49, 58, 149, 204
computer, 142
configuration, viii, 32, 44, 153, 165
conflict, 4
congenital defect, vii, 1, 162, 195
congenital heart disease, 92
congenital malformations, 91
Congress, iv
congruence, 171
connective tissue, 33, 101, 102, 166, 167, 194
consensus, 84, 147, 175
consent, 12
constipation, xi, 49, 139, 141, 144
construction, 33, 35, 36, 46, 48, 49
contamination, 43, 45, 53, 127, 158, 172, 178
contour, 202
contracture, 174, 175
control group, ix, 82, 83, 84, 102
controlled trials, 42, 55, 166, 186, 206
controversial, 10
contusion, 73
conventional inguinal herniotomy, x, 111, 115, 116, 118, 119, 120
conversion rate, 45
COPD, xi, 97, 126, 139, 141, 144, 194, 202
copyright, iv
Copyright, iv, 3, 7, 164, 176, 179, 181

coronary artery disease, 131
coronary heart disease, xi, 126
corpus luteum, 147
correlation, 101, 102, 103, 108
cosmetic, vii, 1, 7, 14, 20, 21, 24, 29
cosmetics, 117
cost, 10, 92, 103, 107, 109, 144, 145, 197
cost effectiveness, 103, 109
costochondral junction, 193
cough, 33, 35, 75, 146
coughing, 59, 64, 70, 162, 164
Cox regression, 167
cross-validation, 97
cryptorchidism, 195, 203
CT scan, 69, 78, 197, 201, 204
cure, 3, 5, 25, 183
cyst, 142, 147
cystic fibrosis, 93

D

daily living, 146
damages, iv
danger, xii, 192
data analysis, 169, 186
data set, 169, 171
database, 128
deaths, 3
debridement, 172
decoupling, 165
defects, xi, xii, 33, 34, 35, 39, 46, 51, 52, 53, 65, 71, 73, 74, 91, 97, 118, 127, 139, 140, 143, 144, 145, 146, 147, 148, 150, 152, 155, 157, 158, 162, 163, 165, 167, 170, 171, 172, 179, 180, 184, 185, 187, 188, 191, 194, 195, 199, 202
deficiency, 75
degenerative joint disease, 141
degradation, 174, 175, 188
dehiscence, 36, 92, 137
deposition, 103, 166
depression, 141

derivatives, 173
dermis, 52, 150, 151, 158, 172, 174, 175, 187
detection, 34, 204
dextrocardia, 72
diabetes, 33, 126, 141
dialysis, 127
diaphragm, vii, 72, 74, 75, 77, 78, 100, 101, 102, 104
diaphragmatic hernia, ix, 71, 72, 73, 74, 77, 78, 79, 80, 81, 82, 94, 95, 96, 97
differential diagnosis, 13, 142
dilation, 180
direct observation, 103
discomfort, 46, 142
diseases, 65, 91, 92, 93, 97, 98, 103, 141, 162
dislocation, 11
disorder, ix, 69, 81, 83, 84, 89
displacement, 62, 66, 67, 68, 75
dissenting opinion, 2
distress, 70, 71, 72
distribution, 102, 128, 167, 168
diverticulitis, 196, 204
dogs, 137
donors, 174
drainage, 120, 133, 162, 185
drawing, 182
drugs, 103, 109
duodenum, 65, 66, 68
durability, 42, 43
dysphagia, 75, 76, 92, 104, 105
dysplasia, 62

E

edema, 102, 126, 135
editors, 25, 79
Ehlers-Danlos syndrome, 165
elastin, 174
elongation, 102
embryogenesis, 195

Index

embryology, 203
emergency, 77, 78, 134, 135, 137, 147, 154, 156
employment, 135
endometriosis, 76
endoscopy, 75
endothelial cells, 174
endotracheal intubation, 20
energy, 92, 95, 97
England, 2
enlargement, 63, 76, 143, 194
enzyme, 103
epidemic, 141
erosion, 40, 41, 52, 76, 105, 163, 168, 182
esophagitis, 92, 102
esophagus, 75, 76, 91, 92, 93, 95, 100, 101, 102, 103, 104, 105, 106, 107, 108
etiology, 2, 4, 25, 78, 101, 192, 194, 197, 202, 203
evidence, xii, 12, 29, 34, 38, 42, 44, 46, 47, 102, 104, 108, 146, 161, 184, 199
evolution, xi, xii, 25, 38, 47, 87, 88, 92, 112, 122, 154, 161
excision, 40, 49
exercise, 92, 171
expertise, 192, 201
exposure, 39, 43, 149, 152, 158
external oblique, 4, 5, 7, 8, 20, 37, 58, 60, 61, 64, 164, 176, 177, 179, 181, 193, 194, 198, 199
extraction, viii, 2, 20, 21, 29

F

fabrication, 175
failure to thrive, 71, 92
families, 102
family history, 10
family members, 10
fascia, vii, xiii, 5, 8, 9, 22, 35, 38, 39, 42, 43, 46, 58, 59, 60, 62, 63, 64, 127, 141, 144, 146, 148, 149, 150, 151, 152, 163, 164, 165, 167, 168, 185, 192, 193, 194, 199, 202
fat, 8, 22, 60, 62, 63, 72, 93, 97, 120, 152, 176, 192, 194, 196, 197, 201
Fata, 79
fear, 13, 23, 121
female rat, 65
femoral hernia, 10, 61, 62, 76, 115
fetus, 147, 148
fever, 59
fiber, 165
fibers, 7, 22, 23, 102, 162, 164, 165, 194
fibrin, 182, 189
fibroblast growth factor, 185
fibroblasts, 174
fibrosis, 76, 93, 101, 102, 120
fixation, xii, 45, 53, 140, 150, 153, 154, 162, 167, 182, 183, 189
flank, 12, 152
flexibility, 197
fluid, 59, 68, 72, 73, 75, 112, 113, 136, 148, 149, 166, 185, 197
Foley catheter, 60
food, 100, 102
foramen, 65, 68, 71, 79
foramen ovale, 71
formation, vii, ix, 2, 7, 13, 18, 35, 39, 45, 49, 50, 57, 68, 69, 102, 103, 120, 147, 151, 154, 165, 166, 168, 171, 172, 173, 174, 182, 185
fractures, 103
France, 81
fresh frozen plasma, 133, 134
fusion, 195

G

gallbladder, 196
gastrectomy, 106
gastric-tube feeding, ix, 82
gastroesophageal reflux, ix, x, 81, 82, 84, 94, 95, 96, 97, 98, 100, 109, 110

gastrointestinal tract, 127, 130
general anesthesia, 147
general surgeon, 33
genetic predisposition, 195
Germany, 125, 128
gestation, 70, 85, 112
gestational age, 83
glue, 182
glycerol, 173
glycol, 173
grading, 188
gravity, 152
growth, ix, 81, 83, 84, 89, 90, 91, 92, 94, 162, 166, 167, 174, 185
growth factor, 166, 185
guidance, 177
guidelines, 29, 35, 36

H

HE, 138
healing, 119, 121, 126, 145, 149, 155
health, 78, 171
health care, 78
heart disease, xi, 92, 126
height, ix, 82, 83, 92
height-for-age (H/A), ix, 82, 83
hematemesis, 77
hematoma, 144, 149, 151, 154, 177, 184
heme, 137
hemostasis, 151
hernia, vii, viii, ix, x, xi, xii, 1, 2, 3, 4, 5, 6, 7, 8, 9, 10, 11, 12, 13, 14, 15, 16, 17, 18, 19, 20, 21, 22, 23, 24, 25, 26, 27, 28, 29, 31, 32, 33, 34, 35, 37, 38, 39, 40, 41, 42, 43, 44, 45, 46, 47, 48, 49, 50, 51, 52, 53, 54, 55, 57, 58, 59, 60, 61, 62, 63, 64, 65, 66, 67, 68, 69, 70, 71, 72, 73, 74, 75, 76, 77, 78, 79, 80, 82, 94, 95, 96, 97, 100, 101, 102, 103, 104, 105, 106, 107, 108, 109, 110, 111, 112, 113, 114, 115, 116, 117, 118, 119, 120, 121, 122, 123, 124, 125, 126, 131, 132, 133, 134, 135, 137,락138, 139, 140, 141, 142, 143, 144, 145, 146, 147, 148, 149, 150, 151, 152, 153, 154, 155, 156, 157, 158, 159, 160, 162, 163, 164, 165, 166, 167, 169, 170, 171, 172, 173, 175, 176, 177, 178, 179, 180, 181, 182, 183, 184, 185, 186, 187, 188, 189, 191, 192, 193, 194, 196, 197, 198, 199, 200, 201, 202, 203, 204, 205, 206
hernia repair, vii, viii, ix, xi, 1, 9, 10, 12, 13, 14, 17, 20, 21, 23, 24, 25, 28, 29, 32, 33, 38, 39, 40, 41, 42, 43, 44, 45, 46, 47, 50, 51, 52, 53, 54, 55, 78, 94, 95, 104, 105, 106, 107, 109, 110, 113, 114, 115, 117, 119, 121, 122, 123, 124, 131, 135, 140, 143, 144, 145, 146, 148, 149, 150, 152, 153, 154, 155, 156, 157, 158, 159, 160, 162, 163, 165, 166, 167, 168, 169, 170, 171, 172, 173, 175, 177, 178, 179, 182, 183, 184, 185, 186, 187, 188, 189, 196, 199, 200, 201, 205, 206
hernia sac, vii, xi, 1, 4, 8, 12, 13, 14, 16, 18, 20, 21, 22, 23, 34, 37, 39, 58, 59, 60, 66, 69, 72, 73, 104, 112, 115, 116, 117, 119, 121, 123, 139, 142, 143, 150, 151, 153, 194, 197, 201
herniated, 60, 62, 66, 67, 68, 72, 73, 74, 75, 77, 78, 91
herniorrhaphy, 25, 27, 28, 29, 60, 61, 110, 119, 123, 157, 160, 187
hiatal hernia, vii, x, 75, 99, 100, 101, 102, 104, 105, 106, 107, 109, 110
hip fractures, 103
history, viii, xi, xii, xiii, 2, 10, 11, 33, 35, 128, 130, 132, 139, 141, 142, 155, 159, 161, 185, 192, 196
hormone, 147, 159
hospitalization, 154
host, 41, 145, 174
human, 52, 135, 158, 172, 174, 175, 183, 186, 187, 188
Hunter, 108

Index

hydrocele, vii, 2, 13, 15, 18, 29, 112, 113, 114, 116, 117, 120
hypersensitivity, 173
hypertension, 71, 82, 90, 130, 132, 141, 149, 160
hypertrophy, xi, 139, 141, 144
hypoplasia, 71, 72, 82, 83, 90, 91, 92, 93
hypotension, 71
hypothesis, ix, 81
hypoxia, 71

I

identification, 24, 200
ileostomy, 38, 47, 48, 49, 50, 127
ileum, 67
iliac crest, 64
imaging modalities, 142
immune function, 174
immune system, 175
immunosuppression, 132
impairments, 91
imperforate anus, 32
implants, 40, 41, 144, 145
incarcerated hernia, 63
incarceration, ix, 3, 8, 35, 38, 57, 62, 71, 72, 76, 100, 113, 135, 140, 142, 146, 147, 148, 172, 192, 196, 197, 198, 202
incidence, vii, viii, 2, 10, 11, 12, 14, 18, 26, 31, 33, 34, 36, 43, 46, 47, 59, 61, 71, 72, 76, 82, 91, 92, 94, 101, 105, 126, 129, 134, 135, 136, 140, 141, 143, 160, 165, 170, 185, 201, 202, 203
incisional abdominal wall hernia, viii, 31
incisional hernia, vii, xi, xii, 33, 34, 39, 40, 42, 43, 45, 51, 52, 53, 69, 77, 79, 80, 102, 125, 126, 132, 133, 134, 136, 137, 138, 157, 158, 161, 162, 163, 165, 166, 167, 168, 169, 170, 171, 172, 182, 184, 185, 186, 187, 206
incisional hernia (IH), xi, 125, 126

individuals, 141, 142, 165, 169, 170, 172, 173, 178
industry, 184
infancy, 24, 25, 72, 96, 112
infants, 6, 7, 8, 9, 25, 26, 28, 62, 85, 86, 87, 88, 89, 91, 92, 94, 95, 97, 112, 122, 140, 155
infarction, 77
infection, 24, 36, 40, 41, 42, 46, 51, 69, 103, 109, 136, 137, 144, 145, 146, 149, 151, 154, 157, 162, 168, 169, 172, 173, 175, 177, 182, 184, 195, 201, 202
inflammation, 66, 67, 102, 173, 182
inflammatory bowel disease, 33, 52
inflammatory cells, 166, 174
informed consent, 12
inguinal, vii, x, xi, 1, 2, 3, 4, 5, 6, 7, 8, 9, 10, 11, 12, 13, 14, 15, 16, 17, 18, 19, 20, 21, 22, 23, 24, 25, 26, 27, 28, 29, 58, 59, 60, 61, 62, 76, 102, 111, 112, 113, 115, 116, 117, 118, 119, 120, 121, 122, 123, 124, 165, 196, 198, 201, 203, 204
inguinal hernia, vii, x, xi, 1, 2, 3, 4, 5, 6, 7, 8, 9, 10, 11, 12, 13, 14, 15, 16, 19, 20, 21, 24, 25, 26, 27, 28, 29, 58, 59, 60, 76, 111, 112, 113, 115, 116, 117, 118, 119, 121, 122, 123, 124, 196, 198, 201, 203, 204
Inguinal hernia, vii, 1, 25, 27, 61, 112, 124
inguinal hernias, 10, 13, 16, 26, 27, 28, 58, 60, 76, 122, 123, 124, 201, 203
inhibitor, 71, 109
injure, 18, 152
injuries, vii, 2, 18
injury, iv, 15, 20, 45, 79, 80, 103, 112, 115, 118, 120, 149, 168, 204
insertion, 71, 162, 163, 172, 173, 174, 176, 177, 182
institutions, 25
integration, xii, 41, 42, 43, 145, 162, 173, 174, 175

integrity, 33, 39, 44, 64, 91, 108, 153, 166, 168, 173
intensive care unit, 109, 130, 134
internal oblique, 5, 23, 37, 61, 164, 165, 176, 177, 179, 180, 193, 194
intervention, viii, 11, 32, 46, 77, 103, 104, 105, 107, 140, 141, 147, 148, 172
intestinal obstruction, 64, 65, 66, 67, 142
intestine, 8, 58, 59, 66, 68, 76, 162, 197
inversion, 124, 152
ipsilateral, 10, 12, 13, 27, 195
irritability, 147
ischemia, 38, 67, 73, 127, 143, 149, 160, 177
issues, 33, 41, 163

J

Japan, 1, 16, 17, 108
jaundice, 162
jejunum, 68
Jordan, 108
jumping, 120

K

K^+, 103
Keloid, 131
kidney, 64, 149

L

laparoscope, 18, 115
laparoscopic cholecystectomy, 160
laparoscopic percutaneous extracorporeal closure (LPEC), vii, 1
laparoscopic surgery, x, 100, 103, 110, 111, 113, 115, 116, 117, 118, 119, 120, 122, 123, 146, 171, 175
laparoscopy, vii, 1, 10, 11, 12, 13, 20, 24, 36, 45, 54, 100, 113, 114, 147, 149, 163, 170, 173, 177, 196, 198, 200, 201

laparotomy, xi, 36, 39, 42, 43, 45, 46, 50, 51, 64, 65, 66, 74, 125, 126, 127, 129, 130, 132, 133, 134, 137, 195, 196, 199
latissimus dorsi, 64
lead, xii, 8, 34, 41, 74, 103, 106, 142, 145, 161, 194, 195, 196
leakage, 127, 131, 136, 148, 149
learning, 6
left-side congenital diaphragmatic hernia, ix, 82
lifestyle changes, 103
ligament, viii, 2, 4, 5, 7, 8, 20, 23, 58, 59, 60, 61, 62, 68, 75, 76, 112, 140
lipoma, 60, 197
liver, 63, 67, 70, 71, 73, 74, 79, 85, 86, 89, 92, 144, 148, 149, 159
liver cirrhosis, 63, 144
liver disease, 148, 149, 159
liver failure, 149
liver transplant, 159
liver transplantation, 159
local anesthesia, 147
local anesthetic, 154
longevity, 166, 183
lordosis, 165
lower esophageal sphincter, 100, 101
lumen, 78
lung disease, 63, 93, 96
lung function, 92, 93
lying, 8, 59, 114, 142, 196, 201

M

macrophages, 98, 174
magnetic resonance, 58
magnetic resonance imaging, 58
majority, 3, 8, 100, 103, 142, 143, 166, 172, 174, 194, 197
malignancy, 132
malnutrition, 33, 69, 92, 95, 149
man, 181

management, x, xi, 26, 27, 35, 38, 49, 54, 74, 92, 95, 97, 100, 103, 104, 108, 109, 127, 133, 139, 140, 148, 188, 203
manipulation, xi, 112, 115, 121, 147, 163, 173
Marx, 136
mass, xi, 63, 64, 65, 66, 68, 93, 97, 113, 126, 128, 130, 132, 134, 142, 143, 194, 195, 197, 198, 201, 204
materials, xii, 39, 40, 41, 44, 115, 145, 161, 162, 163, 168, 169, 173, 174, 183, 188
matrix, 41, 52, 53, 158, 185, 186, 187, 188
matrix metalloproteinase, 185
matter, iv, 144
measurement, 93
measurements, 93, 97
median, xi, 24, 64, 85, 86, 91, 125, 128, 129, 135, 183, 185
mediastinum, vii, 75, 107
medical, 39, 82, 83, 93, 98, 100, 103, 109, 132, 145, 146
medical history, 132
medication, 93
medicine, 104
memory, 41
mental health, 171
mesenchyme, 195
mesenteric vessels, 67
mesentery, 38, 66, 68, 73
meta-analysis, 27, 46, 51, 55, 109, 156, 157, 169, 170, 187, 201
methodology, xii, 38, 161
microorganisms, 40, 144
migration, xii, 75, 91, 105, 107, 140, 154, 195
MMP, 185
models, 84, 102, 167
modifications, 6, 13, 14, 45, 162
morbidity, viii, ix, xi, xiii, 32, 36, 45, 47, 57, 71, 81, 82, 83, 92, 93, 94, 95, 97, 100, 106, 110, 140, 141, 142, 144, 148, 154, 169, 175, 192, 201

morphology, 26
mortality, ix, xi, 57, 62, 70, 72, 78, 110, 126, 135, 140, 141, 142, 148, 154
mortality rate, 62, 72, 141, 142, 148, 154
mortality risk, 70
MRI, 58, 70, 74
mucosa, 103, 104
multivariate analysis, 48, 131, 134
muscle strength, 93
muscles, xii, 4, 20, 22, 23, 37, 74, 92, 101, 102, 163, 164, 165, 167, 173, 176, 177, 179, 180, 191, 195
muscular mass, 93

N

nasogastric tube, 152
nausea, 59, 66, 72, 77
necrosis, 73, 127, 168, 172, 197
negotiating, 120
neonates, 83, 92, 94, 95, 97
neovascularization, 174
nerve, 58, 61, 62, 65
New York, iv
Nissen fundoplication, 100, 104, 105, 109, 110
nitric oxide, 71, 83, 135
nitrite, 63
normal children, 96
nosocomial pneumonia, 109
nutrition, 85, 93
nutritional status, 92

O

obesity, xi, 24, 33, 63, 101, 126, 139, 141, 144, 162, 194, 195, 202
obstruction, viii, ix, xii, xiii, 32, 38, 57, 59, 64, 65, 66, 67, 75, 77, 78, 91, 96, 106, 140, 142, 154, 192, 195, 197, 198, 204
obstructive lung disease, 63

obstructive sleep apnea, 141
oesophageal, 108, 109
OH, 25, 152
old age, 69
omentum, xi, xii, 8, 59, 63, 67, 72, 73, 76, 139, 142, 147, 148, 191, 194, 196, 197
omission, 116
operations, 10, 36, 76, 79, 123, 129, 130, 131, 132, 133, 144
organ, vii, 73, 76, 135, 137, 149, 192, 197
organs, 20, 40, 43, 63, 74, 75, 127, 149, 168, 173, 174, 196
osteogenesis imperfecta, 165
outpatients, 142
overlap, 41, 42, 43, 45, 143, 146, 151, 153, 167, 168, 179, 200
overlay, 150, 175
overweight, 141
overweight adults, 141
oxidation, 137
oxidative stress, 124
oxygen, 92, 137

P

pain, viii, xii, 18, 19, 32, 38, 39, 59, 61, 62, 63, 65, 66, 67, 68, 72, 73, 75, 77, 116, 140, 142, 143, 146, 152, 153, 154, 158, 163, 169, 182, 195, 198, 201, 204
palpation, 20, 23
pancreas, 66, 67
pancreatitis, 127, 181
paracentesis, 148
parallel, 4, 7, 44, 60, 194
parastomal hernia, vii, viii, ix, 31, 32, 33, 34, 35, 36, 37, 38, 39, 40, 41, 42, 43, 44, 45, 46, 48, 49, 50, 51, 52, 53, 54, 55, 69
parents, 12, 24
patent processus vaginalis (PPV), vii, 2
patents, 144
pathogenesis, x, 96, 99, 101, 102

pathology, 35, 128, 197, 201, 202
pathophysiology, x, xii, 99, 102, 161
pectineus, 62
pediatric surgeons, vii, 1, 4, 6, 12, 112, 121
pelvis, 22, 62, 68, 147
penis, 61
percentile, 92
percutaneous extraperitoneal closure, xi, 17, 25, 112, 116, 117, 121, 124
perforation, ix, xi, 38, 52, 57, 67, 72, 73, 76, 105, 126, 127, 128, 130, 131, 132, 194
perfusion, 94, 121, 124, 135
pericardium, 174
perinatal, 85
peristalsis, 108
peritoneal cavity, viii, 9, 32, 42, 74
peritoneal lavage, 74
peritoneum, 13, 14, 18, 61, 70, 72, 116, 117, 118, 119, 120, 151, 167, 174, 193, 196, 199, 200, 201
peritonitis, vii, xi, xiii, 125, 126, 127, 128, 129, 130, 131, 132, 133, 134, 135, 136, 137, 148, 192, 196
permeability, 126
permission, iv, 11, 16, 21, 176, 179, 181, 193
permit, 42, 43
pH, 93, 94, 98, 103
pharynx, 100
Philadelphia, 25, 28
physicians, ix, 57, 197
physics, 38
physiological factors, 33
physiology, 165
pigs, 189
plastics, 51, 157
platform, 128
pleura, 72
PM, 28
pneumonia, 75, 103, 109, 155
polymer, 185

polymers, 41
polyp, 63
polypropylene, 40, 41, 42, 43, 44, 51, 52, 55, 143, 150, 158, 162, 163, 168, 172, 173, 178, 182, 187, 199, 205
polyvinylidene fluoride, 41
population, x, xii, 47, 77, 82, 84, 92, 97, 126, 141, 142, 156, 165, 169, 171, 191, 198
porosity, 173, 174
portal hypertension, 149, 160
portal vein, 68
portraits, 3
postoperative outcome, 49, 128
potassium, 97
potential benefits, 149
pregnancy, 77, 79, 80, 147, 159
premature infant, 140
prematurity, 83
preparation, iv
preterm infants, 95
prevention, 51, 55, 103, 135, 157, 185
primate, 188
principles, 4, 5, 6, 155, 183
probability, 72, 84, 89, 154
probe, 22
prognosis, 70
prolapse, 35, 46, 194
prolapsed, 101
proliferation, 188
prophylactic, ix, 40, 53, 81, 83, 84, 85, 86, 87, 88, 89, 90, 91, 92, 94, 141, 144
prophylactic fundoplication, ix, 81, 83, 84, 85, 86, 87, 88, 89, 90, 91, 92, 94
prophylactic fundoplication group, ix, 82
prophylaxis, 51, 128, 157
prostheses, 144, 145, 178
prosthesis, 51, 52, 54, 61, 106, 144, 146, 151, 153, 157, 163, 167, 174, 180
prosthetic device, 50
prosthetic materials, 39, 168
protection, 173
proteins, 165

proton pump inhibitors, 100, 109
protrusion of abdominal contents, xii, 161
pseudomembranous colitis, 103
PTFE, 51, 52, 110, 157
pubis, 58
pulmonary contusion, 73
pulmonary diseases, 98, 162
pulmonary hypertension, 71, 82, 90
pumps, 103
puncture wounds, 117
pyogenic, 63

Q

quality of life, 38, 103, 171
questionnaire, 104

R

radiography, 58, 69
reactive airway disease, 98
reading, 197
recognition, xi, 112
recommendations, iv, 38, 144, 188
reconstruction, 35, 42, 48, 106, 168, 175, 176, 180, 183, 187, 188, 189
recovery, 15, 18, 19, 63, 73, 115, 149, 177, 201
rectum, 49, 79
rectus abdominis, 36, 37, 46, 50, 59, 63, 163, 164, 167
recurrence, vii, viii, ix, x, xi, xii, xiii, 2, 4, 9, 12, 13, 14, 15, 17, 18, 19, 24, 29, 32, 33, 38, 40, 42, 43, 44, 45, 46, 47, 53, 61, 69, 70, 74, 91, 100, 105, 106, 111, 112, 116, 117, 120, 122, 124, 140, 143, 144, 145, 146, 148, 149, 150, 154, 155, 156, 158, 162, 165, 166, 167, 168, 169, 170, 171, 172, 173, 175, 177, 178, 180, 183, 184, 187, 192, 200, 201
red blood cells, 133, 134
regeneration, 188

regression, 84, 167
regression model, 84, 167
reinforcement, ix, 4, 32, 37, 38, 41, 42, 43, 44, 45, 46, 60, 107, 110, 140, 145, 149, 180
relaxation, 137, 147
relief, 77
repair, vii, viii, ix, xi, xiii, 1, 4, 5, 8, 9, 10, 11, 12, 13, 14, 16, 17, 18, 20, 21, 23, 24, 25, 26, 28, 29, 32, 33, 35, 38, 39, 40, 41, 42, 43, 44, 45, 46, 47, 50, 51, 52, 53, 54, 55, 59, 60, 61, 64, 70, 71, 74, 76, 77, 78, 81, 82, 83, 84, 85, 86, 91, 92, 93, 94, 95, 96, 97, 101, 102, 104, 105, 106, 107, 108, 109, 110, 112, 113, 114, 115, 117, 118, 119, 121, 122, 123, 124, 128, 129, 131, 135, 136, 140, 141, 142, 143, 144, 145, 146, 147, 148, 149, 150, 152, 154, 155, 156, 157, 158, 159, 160, 162, 163, 165, 166, 167, 169, 170, 171, 172, 173, 175, 177, 178, 179, 182, 183, 184, 185, 186, 187, 188, 189, 192, 199, 200, 201, 202, 203, 205, 206
resection, 14, 28, 35, 59, 124, 142, 147, 154, 172, 199
resistance, 42, 173
resolution, 93, 107
resources, 107
respiration, 108, 164
respiratory failure, 92, 93, 97, 155
response, 126, 135, 136, 165, 188
restrictions, 103
retardation, 92
rights, iv
rings, 9, 13, 26
risk, vii, viii, x, xi, 10, 12, 26, 31, 33, 34, 35, 37, 40, 41, 42, 49, 60, 61, 69, 70, 71, 82, 92, 96, 97, 100, 101, 103, 108, 109, 125, 126, 131, 132, 134, 136, 142, 143, 144, 145, 146, 156, 162, 167, 170, 173, 174, 182, 183, 201
risk factors, vii, xi, 49, 125, 126, 132, 134, 136, 156, 162, 182

risks, 20, 144, 162, 173, 182, 183
robotics, 107
routines, 18
rowing, 79

S

safety, 24, 53, 104, 169
SAP, 128
savings, 104
scar tissue, 118, 141, 148
school, 141
sciatica, 65
science, 184
scope, 145, 152
scrotal, 113
scrotum, 4, 22, 61, 112
secretion, 68, 103
seeding, 40, 144
selective sac extraction method (SSEM), viii, 2, 20, 21
sensitivity, 197, 198
sepsis, 33, 137, 169, 172
septic shock, 136
services, iv
sex, 85, 89, 162
shock, 136
shortness of breath, 72
showing, 14, 118, 119
sigmoid colon, 61, 67, 68
signs, 64, 65, 73, 76, 77, 127, 128, 196, 197, 201
silk, 8
silkworm, 4
silver, 63
simple closure, 145
skin, viii, 2, 4, 6, 7, 8, 20, 23, 24, 50, 59, 62, 112, 116, 117, 122, 127, 140, 142, 146, 148, 150, 151, 152, 153, 165, 167, 176, 177, 179, 181
sleep apnea, 141
small intestine, 59, 197

Index

smoking, 126
solution, 35, 40, 120, 186
species, 183
speech, 5
sphincter, 100, 101
Spigelian hernia, xii, 78, 191, 192, 193, 194, 195, 196, 197, 198, 199, 200, 201, 202, 203, 204, 205
spinal cord, 71
spine, 58, 193
spleen, 73, 75, 104
stab wounds, 80
stability, 71
stabilization, 83
standard deviation, 83
starch, 136
state, 55, 117, 122, 192
states, 137
stenosis, 46
stoma, viii, 31, 32, 33, 34, 35, 36, 37, 38, 39, 40, 42, 43, 44, 45, 46, 47, 48, 50, 51, 54, 55, 69, 70, 77
stomach, vii, 66, 67, 68, 72, 73, 75, 92, 100, 101, 103, 104, 107, 196
strangulated hernia, 3
stress, 14, 18, 77, 124
stretching, 35, 39, 196
stroma, 69
structural characteristics, 173
structure, viii, 2, 20, 22, 50, 72, 76, 115, 149
subcutaneous endoscopically assisted ligation (SEAL), vii, 1, 15
subcutaneous tissue, 16, 24, 60, 117, 180
submucosa, 52, 106, 174, 187
substrate, 166, 173, 174, 175
substrates, 166, 173, 174, 175
success rate, 24
supplementation, 202
suppression, 108
suprapubic, 6
surface area, 43, 167

surgical intervention, viii, 11, 32, 46, 100, 103, 104, 105, 107, 140, 141, 147, 148, 172
surgical technique, xi, 110, 112, 126, 183
survival, ix, 79, 81, 82, 84, 88, 90, 91, 126, 129
survival rate, 82
survivors, 44, 71, 72, 82, 83, 91, 95
susceptibility, 108
suture, xii, 8, 13, 14, 16, 17, 18, 19, 28, 38, 39, 60, 65, 105, 106, 112, 115, 116, 117, 118, 119, 120, 121, 127, 130, 131, 133, 140, 143, 150, 151, 152, 153, 154, 156, 158, 160, 162, 166, 167, 179, 182, 183, 185, 199, 200
swelling, 59, 167
symptoms, iv, vii, x, 18, 35, 38, 46, 59, 63, 64, 65, 66, 76, 77, 93, 98, 99, 100, 103, 104, 105, 107, 154, 195, 201
syndrome, 71, 72, 105, 127, 165
synthetic polymers, 41

T

Taiwan, 57, 111
teams, 82, 98
techniques, vii, x, xii, xiii, 1, 13, 29, 36, 38, 40, 42, 43, 45, 46, 49, 110, 112, 115, 116, 117, 121, 136, 162, 163, 169, 177, 182, 183, 185, 192
technologies, 183
tendon, 13
tensile strength, 41, 119, 121, 145, 165, 166
tension, xii, 14, 38, 39, 40, 83, 102, 105, 107, 140, 143, 144, 146, 150, 151, 153, 155, 157, 163, 164, 167, 176
testicle, 4, 196
testing, 93
testis, 22, 23, 112, 113, 204
TGF, 166
therapeutics, 159

therapy, viii, 32, 33, 35, 93, 98, 104, 109, 126, 132, 134, 135, 136
thorax, 70, 72, 73, 74, 101
thrombocyte, 135
time frame, 170
tissue, viii, xii, 8, 16, 22, 24, 32, 33, 39, 41, 44, 74, 77, 101, 116, 119, 120, 127, 135, 141, 143, 145, 148, 151, 156, 162, 163, 165, 166, 167, 168, 173, 174, 175, 177, 179, 180, 184, 188, 194
titanium, 41, 182, 189
torsion, 77
training, 155
transection, 5, 6, 23, 123
transfusion, 133, 135
translation, 176
translocation, 24, 50
transmission, 41
transplant, 149
transplantation, 71, 159, 162
transverse colon, 66, 72
transversus abdominis, 37, 60, 61
trauma, 58, 63, 66, 67, 73, 74, 118, 120, 195
treatment, iv, vii, x, xi, xii, xiii, 2, 3, 4, 5, 7, 20, 25, 27, 45, 48, 49, 50, 52, 78, 79, 83, 84, 91, 96, 98, 99, 100, 103, 104, 105, 106, 112, 121, 124, 126, 133, 135, 136, 137, 138, 143, 152, 158, 161, 166, 169, 171, 172, 183, 184, 186, 189, 192, 201, 202, 203, 204, 205
trial, 29, 46, 48, 49, 55, 103, 106, 109, 110, 123, 136, 143, 156, 158, 159, 160, 182, 183, 185, 200, 205
trisomy, 71
tumors, 63
type 1 collagen, 165
type 2 diabetes, 141

U

UK, 3, 109

ulcerative colitis, 47
ultrasonography, 78, 142, 205
ultrasound, xii, 70, 71, 79, 149, 192, 196, 201
umbilical hernia, xi, 47, 76, 139, 140, 141, 142, 143, 144, 145, 146, 147, 148, 149, 150, 152, 153, 154, 155, 156, 157, 159, 160
uniform, 34, 39
United, 156
United States, 156
urinary retention, 60
urinary tract, 146
urinary tract infection, 146
urine, 59, 63, 152
USA, 31, 99, 139, 152, 161, 191
uterus, 58, 77, 79, 80, 147

V

validation, 97
valsalva, 35
valuation, 25, 123
valve, viii, 32, 44, 84
variables, 85, 128
variations, 102
varieties, 173
vas deferens, 4, 11, 14, 112, 115, 116, 118, 119
vein, 65, 66, 68, 149, 159
ventilation, 71, 83, 94, 134
ventricular septal defect, 72
vertebrae, 100
vessels, vii, 2, 4, 7, 11, 13, 15, 18, 22, 23, 58, 59, 61, 62, 64, 67, 105, 115, 116, 118, 119, 120, 121, 152, 194
viscera, xi, 20, 37, 68, 74, 77, 91, 139, 142, 146, 148, 151
visualization, 10, 12, 15, 19, 79, 150, 152, 153
voiding, 39
volvulus, ix, 57, 66, 67

vomiting, 59, 68, 72, 73, 75, 77, 162

W

walking, 171
Washington, 3
Washington, George, 3
weakness, 5, 69, 74, 141, 148, 149, 162
wear, 154
weight gain, 92, 97
weight loss, 62, 63
Weight-for-height (W/H), ix, 82
western blot, 165
wires, 41
World Health Organization, 83, 141
worldwide, 12
worry, 117
wound dehiscence, 137
wound healing, 126, 145, 149
wound infection, 24, 36, 40, 51, 69, 135, 137, 143, 144, 149, 151, 154, 157, 162, 171, 184, 195, 201

Y

young adults, 123

Z

Z-scores, ix, 82, 83, 87, 88, 89